ECGs for Nurses

Philip Jevon RN BSc (Hons) PGCE
ENB 124 Coronary Care Nursing
Resuscitation Training Officer
Manor Hospital
Walsall

Blackwell
Publishing

© 2003 by Blackwell Science Ltd
a Blackwell Publishing company

Editorial offices:
Blackwell Science Ltd, 9600 Garsington Road, Oxford OX4 2DQ, UK
  Tel: +44 (0) 1865 776868
Blackwell Publishing Inc., 350 Main Street, Malden, MA 02148-5020, USA
  Tel: +1 781 388 8250
Blackwell Science Asia Pty, 550 Swanston Street, Carlton, Victoria 3053, Australia
  Tel: +61 (0)3 8359 1011

First published 2003

Library of Congress Cataloging-in-Publication Data

Jevon, Philip.
  ECGs for nurses / Phil Jevon.
    p. ; cm.
Includes bibliographical references and index.
  ISBN 0-632-05802-1 (pbk. : alk. paper)
  1. Electrocardiography.   2. Arrhythmia–Nursing.
  [DNLM: 1. Electrocardiography–Nurses' Instruction.   2. Arrhythmia–prevention & control–Nurses' Instruction. WG 140 J76w 2003] I. Title.

  RC683.5.E5J48 2003
  616.1'207547–dc21
      2003005902

ISBN 0-632-05802-1

A catalogue record for this title is available from the British Library

Set in 9/12pt Palatino
by SNP Best-set Typesetter Ltd., Hong Kong
Printed and bound in Great Britain using acid-free paper
by MPG Books, Bodmin Cornwall

For further information on Blackwell Publishing, visit our website:
www.blackwellpublishing.com

Contents

Foreword

I am delighted to write this foreword for a new and exciting ECG book for nurses.

Coronary heart disease is among the biggest killers in the country. More than 1.4 million people suffer from angina. 300 000 people have a heart attack every year. More than 110 000 people die of heart problems in England every year (Department of Health 2000).

The risk of death is the highest within the first hour of myocardial infarction and is usually due to arrhythmias (NICE 2002). Arrhythmias are commonly experienced by patients with coronary heart disease (Jowett & Thompson 2003). It is imperative that nurses not only correctly identify arrhythmias, but also appreci-ate their significance and necessary management. This book outlines all arrhythmias in a logical fashion using a five-stage approach to analysis with examples fol-lowed by possible effects on the patient, and finally, treatment. Chapters exploring arrhythmias include the conduction system, principles of monitoring, arrhyth-mias originating in the sinoatrial node, atria, atrioven-tricular junction, ventricles and heart blocks. These chapters will facilitate the development of the practi-tioner's knowledge of arrhythmias by giving concrete examples of application and practice.

The National Service Framework for coronary heart disease (2000) has identified a target for thrombolysis to be administered to patients with a myocardial infarction, without contraindications, within 20 minutes of arrival in hospital. Nurses have an increasingly important role to identify patients in this category as they require urgent attention. These situations require skills in 12 Lead electrocardiogram (ECG) recording and interpretation. *ECGs for Nurses* has two chapters dedicated to 12 Lead ECGs, one exploring recording, and the other, interpretation. It is vital for nurses to review their skills of ECG recording to ensure accuracy and thoroughness and include right-sided leads and posterior leads as, and when, necessary. A systematic approach is used for 12 Lead electrocardiogram analysis and a comprehensive exploration of, for example, myocardial infarction, bundle branch blocks with a variety of ECG examples are included for analysis.

The Nursing and Midwifery Council (2002a) supports lifelong learning for nurses and midwives. It is crucial that practitioners keep abreast of new developments in practice, treatments and technology.

Nurses must take responsibility for their own learning and cultivate an enquiring approach to identify any deficits in personal knowledge or skills that require development (Nursing and Midwifery Council 2002). The code of conduct stipulates that as a registered nurse or midwife, one must maintain professional knowledge and competence (Nursing & Midwifery Council 2002b).

I believe that a knowledgeable nurse, highly skilled in arrhythmia and 12 Lead ECG interpretation and management, who is not afraid to challenge or indeed admit limitations, works with the multidisciplinary team to ensure that patients receive the care they deserve.

I congratulate Philip Jevon for his systematic and very readable approach to ECG interpretation; it is so often seen as a highly complex and incomprehensible topic.

I hope that you enjoy this book as much as I have, and that you also enjoy your lifelong learning journey in pursuit of excellence in care.

Cynthia Curtis
Senior Lecturer
Northumbria University

Department of Health (2000) *National Service Framework for Coronary Heart Disease*. The Stationery Office, London.

Jowett, N.I., Thompson, D.R. (2003) *Comprehensive Coronary Care*, 3rd edn. Baillière Tindall, Edinburgh.

National Institute for Clinical Excellence (2002) *Guidance on the use of drugs for early thrombolysis in the treatment of acute myocardial infarction*. National Institute of Clinical Excellence, London.

Nursing & Midwifery Council (2002a) *Supporting nurses and midwives through lifelong learning*. Nursing & Midwifery Council Publications, London.

Nursing & Midwifery Council (2002b) *Code of professional conduct*. Nursing & Midwifery Council Publications, London.

Acknowledgements

A note of thanks to:

Philips, Medicotest and Medtronic for allowing me to reproduce their images and diagrams. John Hamilton and his colleagues in the Medical Photography Department at the Manor Hospital, Walsall for their help with photographs. Dr Alan Cunnington, Consultant Physician/Cardiologist, Manor Hospital, Walsall for kindly reviewing sections of the text and some of the ECGs. The staff on Coronary Care/Osprey Ward and in Clinical Measurements, Manor Hospital, Walsall for saving ECGs which have been used in this book. Kevin Morris at Aurum Pharmaceuticals for supplying the artwork for the treatment algorithms. Laerdal Medical for supplying four ECG traces.

The Conduction System in the Heart

1

INTRODUCTION

The conduction system in the heart comprises specialised cardiac cells, which initiate and conduct impulses, providing a stimulus for myocardial contraction. Irregularities in the conduction system can cause cardiac arrhythmias and an abnormal electrocardiogram (ECG). An understanding of the conduction system and how it relates to myocardial contraction and the ECG is essential for ECG interpretation.

The aim of this chapter is to understand the conduction system in the heart.

LEARNING OBJECTIVES

At the end of the chapter the reader will be able to:

❏ discuss the basic principles of cardiac electrophysiology;
❏ describe the conduction system in the heart;
❏ describe the normal ECG and how it relates to cardiac contraction;
❏ recognise normal sinus rhythm.

BASIC PRINCIPLES OF CARDIAC ELECTROPHYSIOLOGY

Depolarisation

Depolarisation is the stimulation of the cardiac cell. A change in the cell membrane permeability results in electrolyte concentration changes within the cell. This causes the generation of an electrical current, which spreads to neighbouring cells causing these in turn to depolarise. Depolarisation is represented on the ECG as P waves and QRS complexes.

Repolarisation

Repolarisation is the process by which the cardiac cell returns to its original resting state. Ventricular repolarsiation is represented on the ECG as T waves (atrial repolarisation is not visible on the ECG as it is masked by the QRS complex).

Automaticity

Automaticity is the ability of specialised cardiac cells (automatic or pacemaker cells) to initiate electrical impulses without any external stimulation. The sinus node normally has the fastest firing rate and therefore assumes the role of pacemaker for the heart. If another focus in the heart has a faster firing rate, it will then take over as pacemaker.

Cardiac action potential

Cardiac action potential (Fig. 1.1) is the term used to describe the entire sequence of changes in the

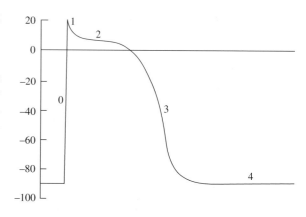

Fig. 1.1 Action potential of cardiac cells (reproduced by kind permission of Scutari Press)

cell membrane potential, from the beginning of depolarisation to the end of repolarisation, i.e. from the beginning of the P wave to the end of the T wave.

Resting cardiac cells have high potassium and low sodium concentrations (140 mmol/l and 10 mmol/l, respectively). This contrasts sharply with extracellular concentrations (4 mmol/l and 140 mmol/l, respectively) (Jowett & Thompson 1995). The cell is polarised and has a membrane potential of −90 mV.

Cardiac action potential results from a series of changes in cell permeability to sodium, calcium and potassium ions. Following electrical activation of the cell, a sudden increase in sodium permeability causes a rapid influx of sodium ions into the cell. This is followed by a sustained influx of calcium ions. The membrane potential is now +20 mV. This is referred to as phase 0 of the action potential.

The polarity of the membrane is now slightly positive. As this is the reverse pattern to that of adjacent cells, a potential difference exists resulting in the flow of electrical current from one cell to the next (Jowett & Thompson 1995).

The cell returns to its original resting state (repolarisation) (phases 1–3); phase 4 ensues. Sodium is

Table 1.1 Phases of the cardiac action potential

Phase	Action
0	Upstroke or spike due to rapid depolarisation
1	Early rapid depolarisation
2	The plateau
3	Rapid repolarisation
4	Resting membrane potential and diastolic depolarisation

Thompson 1997

pumped out and potassium and the transmembrane potential returns to its resting level of −90 mV. Table 1.1 summarises the phases of the cardiac action potential.

Action potential in automatic cells

The action potential in automatic cells differs from that in myocardial cells (Fig. 1.2). Automatic cells can initiate an impulse spontaneously without an external impulse.

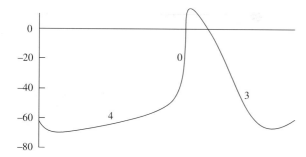

Fig. 1.2 Action potential of automatic or pacemaker cells (reproduced by kind permission of Scutari Press)

Automatic cells can be found in the SA node, AV junction (AV node and Bundle of His), bundle branches and Purkinje fibres. The rate of depolarisation varies between the sites. In normal circumstances, the automatic cells in the SA node have the shortest spontaneous depolarisation time (phase 4) and therefore the quickest firing rate (Julian & Cowan 1993). This is usually about 80 times per minute.

In the atrioventricular junction (AV node and bundle of His), the firing rate is approximately 60 times per minute and in the ventricles 30–40 times per minute. If the SA node firing rate decreases, e.g. a possible complication following an acute inferior myocardial infarction, a subsidiary pacemaker will (hopefully) provide an escape rhythm.

In general, the lower down the conduction system that the pacemaker is sited, the slower the rate, the wider the QRS complex and the less dependable it is (Jowett & Thompson 1995). When an ectopic pacemaker takes over control of the electrical activity in the heart it is denoted by the prefix 'idio', e.g. an idioventricular rhythm is an escape rhythm originating in the ventricles.

THE CONDUCTION SYSTEM IN THE HEART

The heart possesses specialised cells that initiate and conduct electrical impulses resulting in myocardial contraction. These cells form the conduction system (Fig. 1.3) which comprises the following:

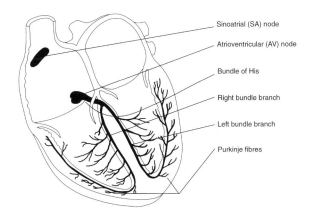

Sinoatrial (SA) node

Atrioventricular (AV) node

Bundle of His

Right bundle branch

Left bundle branch

Purkinje fibres

Fig. 1.3 The conduction system in the heart (reproduced by kind permission of Medicotest, manufacturer of 'blue sensor electrodes')

- *Sinoatrial (SA) node or pacemaker*: situated at the junction of the right atrium and superior vena cava. The blood supply is via the nodal artery which arises from either the right coronary artery (60%) or the left coronary artery (40%) (Jowett & Thompson 1995).

- *AV junction (AV node and bundle of His)*: this acts as a 'bridge' connecting the atria to the ventricles. Blood supply is via the nodal artery which arises from either the right coronary artery (90%) or the left circumflex artery (10%) (Jowett & Thompson 1995).
- *Right and left bundle branches*: the left bundle branch divides into the posterior and anterior fascicles. Blood supply is via the left anterior descending artery (Jowett & Thompson 1995).
- *Purkinje fibres*.

Control of heart rate

The heart rate is controlled by the cardiac centre in the medulla through the autonomic nervous system (Green 1991):

- *Parasympathetic or vagus nerve*: continuous vagal activity or vagal tone acts as a brake on the heart. The greater the vagal activity, the slower the heart rate. Increased vagal tone is often associated with an acute inferior myocardial infarction. If vagal activity diminishes, the heart rate will increase. If the vagal tone is completely blocked, the heart rate would be approximately 150 beats per minute (Green 1991). Atropine blocks the action of the vagus nerve. This causes an increase in heart rate.

- *Sympathetic nerve*: sympathetic nerve activity ('fight and flight') has a positive chronotropic action on the heart, i.e. it increases the heart rate. It is particularly active in periods of emotional excitement, exercise and stress. Beta-blockers shield the heart from sympathetic nerve activity resulting in a decrease in heart rate, blood pressure and myocardial workload.

THE ECG AND ITS RELATION TO CARDIAC CONTRACTION

ECGs relating to the phases of cardiac contraction are shown in Fig. 1.4.

(1) The SA node fires and the electrical impulse spreads across the atria. This results in atrial contraction (P wave).

(2) On arriving at the AV node the impulse is delayed, allowing the atria time to fully contract and eject blood into the ventricles. This brief period of absent electrical activity is represented on the ECG by a straight (isoelectric) line between the end of the P wave and the beginning of the QRS complex. The PR interval represents atrial depolarisation and the impulse delay in the AV node prior to ventricular depolarisation.

(3) The impulse is then conducted down to the ventricles through the bundle of His, right and left bundle branches and Purkinje fibres causing ventricular depolarisation and contraction (QRS complex).

(4) The ventricles then repolarise (T wave).

NORMAL SINUS RHYTHM

Sinus rhythm is the normal rhythm of the heart. The impulse originates in the SA node (i.e. 'sinus') at a regular rate of 60–100 per minute. Each impulse is conducted down the normal pathways to the ventricles

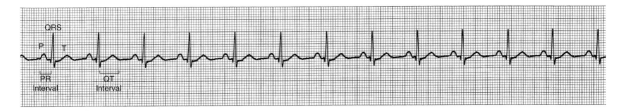

Fig. 1.4 The ECG and its relation to cardiac contraction

without any abnormal conduction delays. It may sometimes present at a cardiac arrest, but without a resultant cardiac output (pulseless electrical activity) (see pages 127–8).

Identifying features on the ECG

- *QRS rate*: 60–100 per min.
- *QRS rhythm*: regular.
- *QRS complexes*: normal width and morphology.
- *P waves*: present and of constant morphology.
- *Relationship between P waves and QRS complexes*: each P wave is followed by a QRS complex and each QRS complex is proceeded by a P wave. PR interval normal and constant.

CHAPTER SUMMARY

The conduction system in the heart comprises specialised cardiac cells, which initiate and conduct impulses, providing a stimulus for myocardial contraction.

The chapter has provided an overview to the conduction system. The basic principles of cardiac electrophysiology have been discussed. The conduction system has been described together with how the ECG relates to cardiac contraction.

REFERENCES

Green, J. (1991) *An Introduction to Human Physiology*. Oxford Medical Publications, Oxford.

Jowett, N.I. & Thompson, D.R. (1995) *Comprehensive Coronary Care*, 2nd edn. Scutari Press, London.

Julian, D. & Cowan, J. (1993) *Cardiology*, 6th edn. Baillière, London.

Thompson, P. (1997) *Coronary Care Manual*. Churchill Livingstone, London.

Principles of Cardiac Monitoring

2

INTRODUCTION

Cardiac monitoring is one of the most valuable diagnostic tools in modern medicine. It is essential if disorders of the cardiac rhythm are to be recognised. It can help with diagnosis and can alert healthcare staff to changes in the patient's condition.

Cardiac monitoring must be meticulously undertaken. Potential consequences of poor technique include misinterpretation of cardiac arrhythmias, mistaken diagnosis, wasted investigations and mismanagement of the patient (Jevon 2000).

The aim of this chapter is to understand the principles of cardiac monitoring.

LEARNING OBJECTIVES

At the end of the chapter the reader will be able to:

❏ list the indications for cardiac monitoring;
❏ state the common features of a cardiac monitor;
❏ describe the positioning of ECG electrodes;
❏ discuss the rationale for selecting particular ECG monitoring leads;
❏ describe the procedure for cardiac monitoring;
❏ discuss the problems associated with cardiac monitoring;
❏ outline what the ECG trace records;
❏ outline the principles of exercise testing.

INDICATIONS FOR CARDIAC MONITORING

Cardiac monitoring (Fig. 2.1) is required in a variety of clinical situations including:

- chest pain;
- myocardial infarction;
- shock;
- heart failure;
- palpitations;
- history of syncope;
- during CPR.

Jevon 2002

COMMON FEATURES OF A CARDIAC MONITOR

The bedside cardiac monitor (Fig. 2.2) or oscilloscope provides a continuous display of the patient's ECG and has the following common features:

- *Screen for displaying the ECG trace*, a dull/bright switch can be adjusted if the screen is too light or too dark.

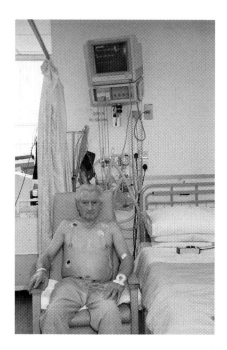

Fig. 2.1 Cardiac monitoring

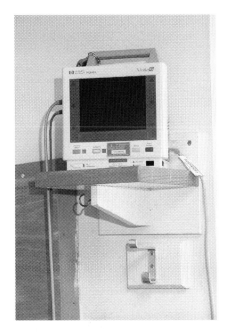

Fig. 2.2 Bedside cardiac monitor

- *ECG printout facility*, to record cardiac arrhythmias (invaluable for both diagnosis and record keeping purposes).
- *Heart rate counter*, to calculate the heart rate (counts the QRS complexes).
- *Monitor alarms*, to alert the healthcare professional to changes in heart rate to outside pre-set limits. Some cardiac monitors can identify important cardiac arrhythmias and changes in the ST segment, and alarm accordingly.
- *Lead select switch*, to select the desired monitoring lead, e.g. lead II.
- *ECG gain*, to alter the size of the ECG complex. If it is set too low or too high the ECG trace can become unrecognisable, either too small or distorted (Fig. 2.3), leading to the possibility of misinterpretation.

POSITIONING OF ECG ELECTRODES
The correct positioning of ECG electrodes is crucial for obtaining accurate information from any monitoring lead (Jacobson 2000). Whether a three or a five ECG

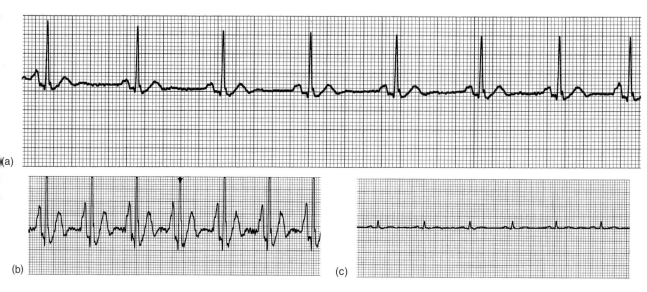

Fig. 2.3 Effects of incorrect ECG gain setting. (a) 10 mm/1 mV – standard setting; ECG complexes adequate size. (b) 40 mm/1 mV – ECG complexes too large; cardiac monitor mistook the P and T waves for QRS complexes resulting in continuous false-high heart rate alarms. (c) 2 mm/1 mV – ECG complexes too small; cardiac monitor did not recognise QRS complexes resulting in continuous false asystole alarms. Also difficulties may be encountered interpreting cardiac arrhythmias when the gain is set too low

cable monitoring system is used will depend upon the patient, the desired monitoring lead(s), local protocols and manufacturer's recommendations.

Three ECG cable system

The standard positioning of ECG electrodes when using a three ECG cable monitoring system is:

- red ECG cable: below the right clavicle;
- yellow ECG cable: below the left clavicle;
- green ECG cable: left lower thorax/hip region.

This electrode position enables the monitoring of lead II. When establishing cardiac monitoring during cardiopulmonary resuscitation (CPR), it is recommended to slightly modify this position: red ECG cable on the right shoulder, yellow ECG cable on the left shoulder and green ECG cable on the left abdominal wall; the precordium should be left unobstructed so as not to hinder defibrillation if it is required (Resuscitation Council UK 2000).

Some clinical areas prefer to monitor on MCL1 (modified chest lead 1, i.e. V1) as recommended by Marriott (1988). The positioning of ECG electrodes is:

- black ECG cable: right shoulder;
- red ECG cable: left shoulder;
- yellow ECG cable: 4th intercostal space, just to the right of the sternum, i.e. corresponding to V1.

Five ECG cable system

Cardiac monitoring using a five ECG cable system is becoming more popular. The main advantage of this system is that different ECG leads can be monitored simultaneously. This is particularly useful when analysing cardiac arrhythmias as it provides an alternative view of the waveform. The standard positioning for ECG electrodes is illustrated in Fig. 2.4 and is as follows:

- RA (red ECG cable): below the right clavicle;
- LA (yellow ECG cable): below the left clavicle;
- RL (black ECG cable): right lower thorax/hip region;

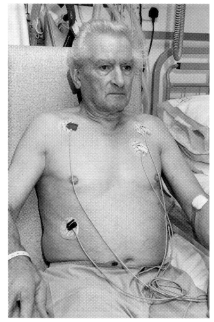

Fig. 2.4 Suggested ECG electrode placement when using a five cable monitoring system

- LL (green ECG cable): left lower thorax/hip region;
- (white ECG cable): on the chest in the desired V position, usually V1 (MCL1, 4th intercostal space just right of the sternum).

Jacobson 2000

EASI 12 lead ECG monitoring

The conventional 12 lead ECG using ten electrodes attached to the limbs and chest is recognised as the current medical standard for the identification, analysis and confirmation of many cardiac abnormalities including cardiac arrhythmias and cardiac ischaemia/infarction.

If 12 lead ECG monitoring is undertaken on a continual basis, the benefits include:

- facilitating the accurate recognition of cardiac arrhythmias;
- enabling the monitoring of the mid-precordial leads which is particularly important for the detection and management of ischaemia;

- enabling the recording of *transient* ECG events of particular diagnostic or therapeutic importance;
- enabling the differentiation between post-PTCA ischaemia and occlusion.

Unfortunately the use of a conventional 12 lead ECG system using ten electrodes for continuous cardiac monitoring is cumbersome and generally not practical in the clinical area.

However, the EASI system, a new concept in 12 lead ECG monitoring, requires the use of only five electrodes:

- *E* electrode on the lower sternum at the level of the fifth intercostal space
- *A* on the left midaxillary line on the same level as the E electrode
- *S* electrode on the upper sternum
- *I* on the right midaxillary line on the same level as the E electrode

A fifth ground electrode can be placed anywhere. The system is illustrated in Fig. 2.5.

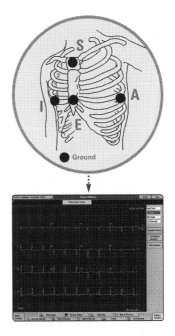

Fig. 2.5 EASI 12 lead ECG monitoring system (reproduced by kind permission of Philips)

The EASI system for 12 ECG (Philips) monitoring using only five electrodes is less cumbersome and more practical than the standard ten electrode system. It is therefore more comfortable for the patient. In addition it will not interfere with such procedures as cardiac auscultation, CPR, defibrillation and echocardiography.

SELECTION OF ECG MONITORING LEADS

When undertaking cardiac monitoring to diagnose cardiac arrhythmias or to detect changes in the cardiac axis, it is important to select an ECG monitoring lead that clearly displays atrial and ventricular activity. The R wave configuration should be at least double the amplitude of the T wave, so that the heart rate will be accurately displayed and computer rhythm analysis will be correct (Thompson 1997).

Lead II provides upright positive waveforms with good visualisation of the P waves. It is used for analysing atrial arrhythmias, differentiating between atrial and junctional arrhythmias, AV blocks and atrial pacing. It is recommended during cardiopulmonary resuscitation. Lead II can be viewed using either of the above ECG electrode positions.

MCL1 (modified chest lead, V1) enables differentiation between ventricular and supraventricular arrhythmias and identification of bundle branch blocks (Meltzer *et al.* 1983). However, it does not enable the recognition of changes in the cardiac axis. MCL1 can be viewed using the ECG electrode position described for the five ECG cable monitoring system or with a modified ECG electrode position for using a three ECG cable system.

PROCEDURE TO ESTABLISH CARDIAC MONITORING

A suggested procedure to establish cardiac monitoring is as follows:

(1) Explain the procedure to the patient.
(2) Clean any greasy areas with a mild soap (do not use alcohol wipes).
(3) Dry the skin. This will help the ECG electrodes to adhere to the skin.

(4) Shave off any excess hair. This will help ensure better contact and also make it less uncomfortable for the patient when removing the ECG electrodes (Perez 1996a).

(5) Gently rub the skin with some gauze (Fig. 2.6). Mild abrasion of the skin will reduce impedance between the skin and electrode, thus reducing interference (Thompson 1997).

(6) Check the ECG electrodes (Fig. 2.7). They should be in date and still moist, not dry.

(7) Remove the protective backing from the ECG electrodes and expose the gel disc (Fig. 2.8).

(8) Apply the ECG electrodes to the patient's chest following locally agreed protocols. The electrodes should lie flat. If the electrodes have an offset connector (to absorb tugs) these should be pointed towards the ECG cables.

(9) Smooth down the adhesive area with a circular motion (Fig. 2.9). Avoid pressing on the gel disc itself as this may result in a decrease in electrode conductivity and adherence (Thompson 1997).

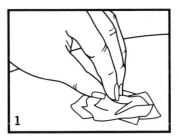

Fig. 2.6 Setting up cardiac monitoring: gently rub the skin (reproduced by kind permission of Medicotest, manufacturer of 'blue sensor electrodes')

(10) Attach the ECG cables to the electrodes (Fig. 2.10). (**NB** If 'snap-on' ECG cables are being used with central stud electrodes, connect them up before application to the patient's skin.)

(11) Switch the cardiac monitor on and select the required monitoring ECG lead.

(12) Ensure the ECG trace is clear. Rectify any difficulties encountered (see below).

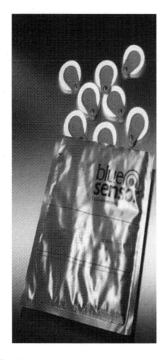

Fig. 2.7 ECG electrodes (reproduced by kind permission of Medicotest, manufacturer of 'blue sensor electrodes')

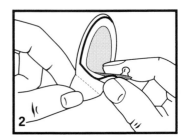

Fig. 2.8 Setting up cardiac monitoring: remove the protective backing from the ECG electrode (reproduced with kind permission by Medicotest, manufacturer of 'blue sensor electrodes')

(13) Set the alarms within safe parameters following locally agreed protocols and appropriate to the patient's clinical condition.

(14) Anchor the ECG cables. They should not be allowed to pull on the ECG electrodes.

(15) Position the cardiac monitor so it is clearly visible.

(16) Document in the patient's notes that cardiac monitoring has commenced and the ECG rhythm identified.

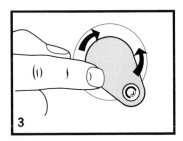

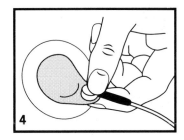

Fig. 2.9 Setting up cardiac monitoring: smooth down the adhesive area with a circular motion. Avoid pressing down in the centre of the ECG electrode because this may disturb the gel column underneath (reproduced by kind permission of Medicotest, manufacturer of 'blue sensor electrodes')

Fig. 2.10 Setting up cardiac monitoring: attach the cables to the electrodes (reproduced by kind permission of Medicotest, manufacturer of 'blue sensor electrodes')

(17) Regularly monitor the electrode sites for signs of allergy – redness, itching and erythema.

Adapted from Jevon 2000

Telemetry

Telemetry (Fig. 2.11) is a convenient method of monitoring the ECG while the patient is mobilising.

ECG electrodes are connected to a small portable transmitter, which the patient carries around in a pyjama pocket or pouch.

The radio signals are transmitted to a central console (normally on CCU) (Fig. 2.12) where any important cardiac arrhythmias can be identified. The advantage of this system is that patients can be mobilised in the

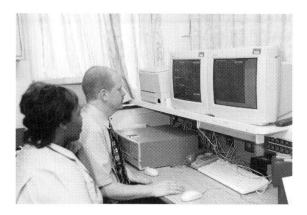

Fig. 2.12 Central console

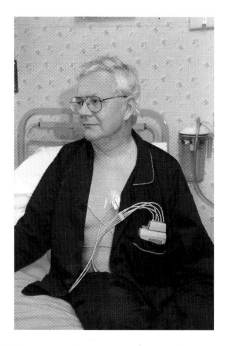

Fig. 2.11 Telemetry monitoring

early period following a myocardial infarction yet still benefit from close cardiac monitoring (Jowett & Thompson 1995). It also frees up monitored CCU beds (Thompson 1997).

Ambulatory cardiac monitoring (24-hour tape)

There are limitations to ECG monitoring when investigating paroxysmal cardiac arrhythmias (Kennedy 1992). To overcome these, ambulatory cardiac monitoring has been developed (Petch 1985).

Ambulatory cardiac monitoring is designed to identify transient disturbances in the ECG rhythm, rate and conduction, together with any associated symptoms (DiMarco & Philbrick 1990). It can help to assess the effectiveness of anti-arrhythmic drug therapy, detect ischaemia and determine prognosis (Mickley 1994).

The patient is asked to continue with normal daily activities. A patient diary should be kept and any episodes of pain, dizziness, palpitations, syncope etc., together with exact timings, should be recorded. Some machines have an 'event marker' button which the patient can press at the onset of symptoms.

A typical 24-hour tape will record 100 000 QRS complexes for analysis. Fortunately, high-speed electrocardioscanners are able to replay the tape in a matter of minutes (Jowett & Thompson 1995). Areas of interest can be printed out, particularly ECG strips during periods when the patient experienced symptoms.

Best practice – ECG monitoring

- Ensure adequate skin preparation.
- Use ECG electrodes that are in date with moist gel sponge.
- Position ECG electrodes and select monitoring lead following locally agreed protocols.
- Set cardiac monitor alarms according to the patient's clinical condition.
- Ensure the ECG trace is accurate.
- Ensure the cardiac monitor is visible.

PROBLEMS ASSOCIATED WITH CARDIAC MONITORING

There are numerous problems associated with cardiac monitoring, some are due to the limitations of the monitoring system itself whereas others are due to poor technique (Meltzer *et al*. 1983). Potential problems that may be encountered are described below.

The 'flat line' trace

(Check the patient!) The most likely cause is mechanical. Check that:

- the correct ECG monitoring lead is selected (usually lead II);
- the ECG gain is set correctly;
- the electrodes are in date and the gel sponge is moist, not dry;
- the ECG cables are properly connected to the electrodes;
- the ECG cables are not broken and are plugged into the monitor.

Poor quality ECG trace

If the ECG trace quality is poor, check:

- all the connections;
- the brightness display;
- the electrodes are in date and that the gel sponge is moist, not dry (Perez 1996a);
- the electrodes are properly attached.

If there are still difficulties obtaining a clear ECG trace, wiping the skin with an alcohol swab may help. If the patient is sweating profusely, the application of a small amount of tincture benzoin to the skin, leaving it to dry before applying the electrodes, is recommended (Jowett & Thompson 1995). As electrodes tend to dry out after about three days, they should be changed at least that often, though every 24 hours may be optimum to maintain skin integrity (Perez 1996a).

Voluntary patient movement artefact or wandering ECG baseline

Voluntary patient movement artefact or wandering ECG baseline (ECG trace going up and down) (Fig. 2.13) is usually caused by patient movement, particularly by respiration. If respiration is the cause and the problem is not transient, reposition the electrodes away from the lower ribs (Meltzer *et al.* 1983). If it occurs in obese patients, it is difficult to correct.

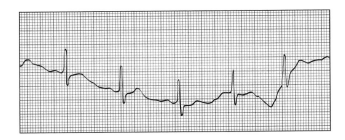

Fig. 2.13 Wandering baseline (reproduced by kind permission of Medicotest, manufacturer of 'blue sensor electrodes')

Involuntary patient movement artefact

Involuntary patient movement artefact is usually caused by a tremor, e.g. if the patient is cold or nervous (Fig. 2.14). The patient should be reassured and kept warm. If the patient has a tremor associated with Parkinson's disease, very little can be done to remedy the artefact.

Electrical interference

Electrical interference, e.g. from bedside infusion pumps, can cause a 'fuzzy' appearance on the ECG trace. Remove the source of the interference if possible.

Loose electrode

A wandering baseline, together with sudden breaks in the signal (Fig. 2.15), often indicates a loose electrode. Causes include incorrect positioning, e.g. over a joint, and poor electrode site, e.g. hairy skin or dry, not moist electrode.

Small ECG complexes

Sometimes the ECG complexes may be too small and unrecognisable. Possible causes include pericardial effusion, obesity and hypothyroidism. However,

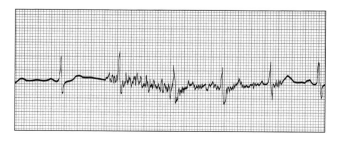

Fig. 2.14 Artefact caused by patient tremor (reproduced by kind permission of Medicotest, manufacturer of 'blue sensor electrodes')

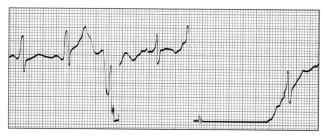

Fig. 2.15 Loose electrode (reproduced by kind permission of Medicotest, manufacturer of 'blue sensor electrodes')

sometimes a technical problem is the cause (Fig. 2.3). Check that the ECG gain is correctly set and the desired ECG monitoring lead has been selected; repositioning the electrodes or selecting another ECG monitoring lead sometimes helps.

Incorrect heart rate display

If the ECG complexes are too small, a false-low heart rate may be displayed. Large T waves, muscle movement and interference can be mistaken for QRS complexes resulting in a false-high heart rate being displayed. The nurse must be alert to the possibility of inaccurate heart rate readings, especially those that might be caused by poor electrode contact and interference (Ren *et al.* 1998). To minimise the potential for inaccuracies, a good quality ECG trace should be obtained.

False alarms

Frequent false alarms will undermine the rationale for setting alarms and will cause undue anxiety for the patient. It is important to ensure that the alarms are correctly and appropriately set. An accurate ECG trace will reduce the frequency of false alarms. A poor connection (Fig. 2.16) can also lead to false alarms.

Skin irritation

ECG electrodes can cause skin irritation. The electrode sites should be regularly examined for redness, itching and erythema. If the patient's skin appears irritated, select another site for electrode placement (Paul & Hebra 1998). If necessary, use hypoallergenic ECG electrodes (Thompson 1997).

PRINCIPLES OF EXERCISE TESTING

Exercise stress testing, first introduced in the 1940s (Master *et al.* 1942), has traditionally been used for the diagnosis of coronary artery disease. However, it is now equally important in the assessment of patients with known disease (Detry & Fox 1996).

It provides an accurate physiological evaluation of coronary flow reserve, which, in terms of prognosis,

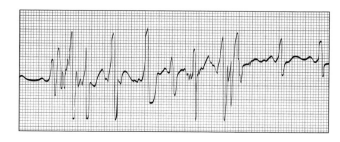

Fig. 2.16 Poor electrode connection (reproduced by kind permission of Medicotest, manufacturer of 'blue sensor electrodes')

becomes more significant than simply the number of anatomical lesions (Detry & Fox 1996).

The main aims of exercise testing are to:

- provoke symptoms, e.g. chest pain and dyspnoea;
- identify ECG changes associated with progressive workload;
- determine maximum workload;
- assess prognosis.

Jowett & Thompson 1995

Generally the early onset of angina with significant and widespread ST depression, slow recovery and a poor blood pressure response are indicative of severe coronary artery disease (Jowett & Thompson 1995).

There are numerous exercise protocols available for diagnostic and prognostic assessment during exercise testing (Detry & Fox 1996). However, the Bruce protocol (Bruce *et al*. 1963) is the most widely used (Detry & Fox 1996). It is suitable for routine use and produces a rapid increase in progressive workload (Jowett & Thompson 1995). For patients with known coronary artery disease, the slower Naughton protocol (Naughton *et al.* 1964) may be better suited (Jowett & Thompson 1995).

Contraindications to exercise testing include unstable angina, severe hypertension, anaemia, electrolyte imbalances and serious cardiac arrhythmias (Jowett & Thompson 1995). As life-threatening cardiac arrhythmias, e.g. ventricular fibrillation, can occur during the test (Irving *et al.* 1977), it is important to ensure that adequate resuscitation facilities are available. National guidelines are available when undertaking exercise testing without direct medical supervision (British Cardiac Society 1993).

CHAPTER SUMMARY

This chapter has provided an overview to the principles of cardiac monitoring. The indications for cardiac monitoring, common features of a cardiac monitor, ECG electrode placement, procedure for cardiac monitoring together with problems associated and what the ECG trace records, have been discussed.

Cardiac monitoring must be meticulously undertaken. Consequences of poor technique could include misinterpretation of cardiac arrhythmias, mistaken diagnosis, wasted investigations and mismanagement of the patient.

REFERENCES

British Cardiac Society (1993) Guidelines on exercise testing when there is not a doctor present. *British Heart Journal* **70**: 488.

Bruce, R., Blackmon, J., Jones, J. & Strait, G. (1963) Exercise testing in adult normal subjects and cardiac patients. *Pediatrics* **32**: 742–56.

Detry, J. & Fox, K. (1996) Exercise testing, in Julian, D., Camm, A., Fox, K. *et al.* (eds) *Diseases of the Heart*, 2nd edn. W.B. Saunders, London.

DiMarco, J. & Philbrick, J. (1990) Use of ambulatory electrocardiographic (Holter) monitoring. *Annals of Internal Medicine* **113**: 53–68.

Irving, J., Bruce, R. & de Rouen, T. (1977) Variations in and significance of systolic pressure during maximal exercise (treadmill) testing. *American Journal of Cardiology* **39**: 841–8.

Jacobson, C. (2000) Optimum bedside cardiac monitoring. *Progress in Cardiovascular Nursing* **15**(4): 134–7.

Jevon, P. (2000) Cardiac monitoring. *Nursing Times* **96**(23): 43.

Jevon, P. (2002) *Advanced Cardiac Life Support*. Butterworth Heinemann, Oxford.

Jowett, N.I. & Thompson, D.R. (1995) *Comprehensive Coronary Care*, 2nd edn. Scutari Press, London.

Kennedy, H. (1992) Importance of the standard electrocardiogram in ambulatory (Holter) electrocardiography. *American Heart Journal* **123**: 1660–77.

Marriott, H. J. L. (1988) *Practical Electrocardiography*, 8th edn. Williams & Wilkins, London.

Master, A., Friedman, R. & Dack, S. (1942) The electrocardiogram after standard exercise as a functional test of the heart. *American Heart Journal* **24**: 777–93.

Meltzer, L.E., Pinneo, R. & Kitchell, J.R. (1983) *Intensive Coronary Care: A Manual for Nurses*, 4th edn. Prentice Hall, London.

Mickley, H. (1994) Ambulatory ST segment monitoring after myocardial infarction. *British Heart Journal* **71**: 113–14.

Naughton, J., Ballke, B. & Nagle, F. (1964) Refinements in methods of evaluation and physical conditioning before and after myocardial infarction. *American Journal of Cardiology* **14**: 837–43.

Paul, S. & Hebra, J. (1998) *The Nurse's Guide to Cardiac Rhythm Interpretation*. W.B. Saunders, London.

Perez, A. (1996a) Cardiac monitoring: mastering the essentials. *Registered Nurse* **59**(8): 32–9.

Perez, A. (1996b) ECG electrode placement: a refresher course. *Registered Nurse* **59**(9): 29–31.

Petch, M. (1985) Lessons from ambulatory electrocardiography. *British Medical Journal* **291**: 617–18.

Ren, Y., Yang, L. & Hu, P. (1998) Analysis of influencing factors on ECG monitoring. *Shanxi Nursing Journal* **12**(5): 213–14.

Resuscitation Council UK (2000) *Advanced Life Support Manual*, 4th edn. Resuscitation Council UK, London.

Thompson, P. (1997) *Coronary Care Manual*. Churchill Livingstone, London.

ECG Interpretation of Cardiac Arrhythmias

INTRODUCTION

Cardiac arrhythmia literally means total lack of rhythm. However, any cardiac rhythm that deviates from the normal sinus rhythm, regardless of the rhythm or whether it is due to a disturbance in impulse formation or impulse conduction, can be classified as a cardiac arrhythmia.

Accurate ECG interpretation of cardiac arrhythmias is essential to ensure the most appropriate management. A systematic approach to ECG interpretation of cardiac arrhythmias is therefore paramount.

The aim of this chapter is to understand ECG interpretation of cardiac arrhythmias.

LEARNING OBJECTIVES

At the end of the chapter the reader will be able to:

❏ list the mechanisms of cardiac arrhythmias;
❏ discuss the classification of cardiac arrhythmias;
❏ describe a five-stage approach for ECG interpretation of cardiac arrhythmias.

MECHANISMS OF CARDIAC ARRHYTHMIAS

There are several mechanisms that can lead to cardiac arrhythmias. Each will now be discussed.

Altered automaticity

Automaticity is the term used to describe the inherent ability of automatic or pacemaker cells to initiate electrical impulses. Altered automaticity can lead to changes in the rate of impulse generation by the SA node, e.g. sinus bradycardia and sinus tachycardia. It is caused by either an increase in autonomic nerve activity or by SA node disease.

If the SA node rate falls or if its impulses are blocked, another group of automatic cells lower down in the conduction system may then take over as pacemaker of the heart, resulting in an escape rhythm.

Enhanced automaticity

Enhanced automaticity may also cause arrhythmias. Causes of enhanced automaticity include increased sympathetic activity, myocardial ischaemia, digoxin toxicity, drugs, electrolyte imbalances, hyperthermia, hypoxia, hypercapnia and acidosis.

Re-entry

The re-entry mechanism is the most common cause of clinically significant cardiac arrhythmias including ventricular fibrillation and most cases of ventricular tachycardia (Tonkin 1997). The re-entry mechanism is caused by a self-perpetuating 'circus movement' of the cardiac impulse (Fig. 3.1).

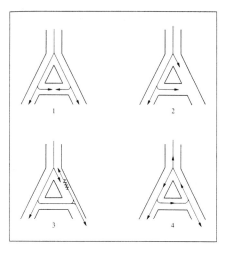

Fig. 3.1 Re-entry causative mechanism of cardiac arrhythmias (reproduced by kind permission of Scutari Press)

The re-entry mechanism requires:

- *non-uniform refractoriness*: this can create an area of unidirectional block;

- *slow conduction*: the conduction time over the re-entry circuit should exceed the longest refractory period of any point in the circuit.

Julian & Cowan 1993

AV nodal re-entrant tachycardia is the commonest cause of paroxysmal regular narrow complex tachycardia (Esberger *et al.* 2002). AV re-entrant tachycardias can occur owing to the presence of an additional pathway, other than the AV junction, connecting the atria and the ventricles, e.g. bundle of Kent (Wolff–Parkinson–White syndrome). This accessory conduction pathway allows the atrial impulse to bypass the AV junction and activate the ventricles prematurely (ventricular pre-excitation) (Esberger *et al.* 2002).

Triggered activity

Triggered activity requires a preceding stimulus to initiate depolarisation – afterdepolarisations are oscillations in the transmembrane potential that are induced by the preceding action potential (Tonkin 1997). Arrhythmias caused by triggered activity include benign ventricular ectopics, torsades de pointes and ventricular fibrillation (Tonkin 1997).

Reperfusion

Reperfusion arrhythmias can occur following spontaneous or drug-induced thrombolysis or coronary angiography (Tonkin 1997). The duration and severity of ischaemia are thought to be key contributory factors.

There appear to be two distinct time-related mechanisms for reperfusion arrhythmias. Immediately following reperfusion, the 're-entry' mechanism, which can precipitate ventricular fibrillation, is significant. 'Triggered activity' and 'enhanced automaticity' are later mechanisms for reperfusion arrhythmias.

Conduction disturbances

Conduction disturbances or AV block (slowing down or complete blocking of an impulse) can occur within the AV junction or bundle branches.

AV block complicates 10% of myocardial infarctions (Jowett & Thompson 1995). Conduction disturbances in the AV junction are usually associated with inferior myocardial infarction and those in the bundle branches with anterior myocardial infarction.

CLASSIFICATION OF CARDIAC ARRHYTHMIAS

Cardiac arrhythmias can be classified into one of two groups: those that result from a disturbance in impulse formation or those that result from a disturbance in impulse conduction (Meltzer *et al.* 1983) (cardiac arrhythmias are discussed in this book according to this classification).

Although this general classification is helpful, it does have limitations as some arrhythmias may result from a disturbance both in impulse formation and conduction.

Arrhythmias resulting from a disturbance in impulse formation

Cardiac arrhythmias that result from a disturbance in impulse formation can be categorised according to their site of origin and mechanism of disturbance:

Site of origin

- *SA node*: sinus rhythms, e.g. sinus bradycardia, sinus arrest.
- *Atria*: atrial rhythms, e.g. atrial ectopics, atrial fibrillation.
- *AV junction*: junctional rhythms, e.g. junction tachycardia.
- *Ventricles*: ventricular rhythms, e.g. ventricular premature beats, ventricular tachycardia.

Mechanism

- Tachycardia > 100 beats/min.
- Bradycardia < 60 beats/min.
- Premature contractions.
- Flutter.
- Fibrillation.

Arrhythmias resulting from a disturbance in impulse conduction

Cardiac arrhythmias that result from a disturbance in impulse conduction refer to an abnormal delay or block of the impulse at some point along the conduction system. They are traditionally categorised according to the site of the defect:

- SA node blocks, e.g. SA block.
- AV blocks, e.g. 1st, 2nd, 3rd degree AV block.
- Intraventricular blocks, e.g. bundle branch blocks.

FIVE-STAGE APPROACH TO ECG INTERPRETATION OF CARDIAC ARRHYTHMIAS

A suggested five-stage approach to ECG interpretation of cardiac arrhythmias is:

(1) Estimate the QRS rate.
(2) Ascertain whether the QRS rhythm is regular or irregular.
(3) Determine whether the QRS complexes are of normal and constant morphology.
(4) Establish whether P waves are present and are of normal and constant morphology.
(5) Examine the relationship between P waves and QRS complexes.

It must be emphasised that displays and ECG printouts from cardiac monitors are suitable for interpreting cardiac arrhythmias only and not for analysis of ST segment changes and more sophisticated ECG interpretation (Resuscitation Council UK 2000). Wherever possible, a 12 lead ECG should be recorded, as this may provide additional diagnostic information.

Each of the five stages for ECG interpretation of cardiac arrhythmias will now be described in turn.

QRS rate

Estimate the QRS rate by counting the number of large (1 cm) squares between two adjacent QRS complexes and dividing the result into 300 (caution if the QRS rate is irregular). For example, the QRS rate in Fig. 3.2 is about 75/min.

An alternative method is to count the number of QRS complexes in a defined number of seconds and then calculate the rate per minute. For example, if there are 12 QRS complexes in a 10 second strip, then the ventricular rate is 72/min (12×6).

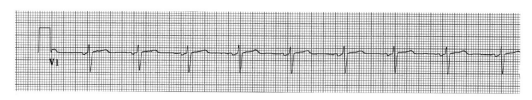

Fig. 3.2 Suggested method for estimating the QRS rate (regular QRS rhythm): divide the number of large squares between two adjacent QRS complexes into 300, i.e. 300/4.2–75/min

- Normal QRS rate: 60–100/min.
- Slow QRS rate (bradycardia): < 60/min.
- Fast QRS rate (tachycardia): > 100/min.

NB A pulse rate of 50 may be 'normal' in some patients and one of 70 may be abnormally slow in other patients.

QRS rhythm

Ascertain whether the QRS rhythm is regular or irregular. Using an adequate length of rhythm strip, carefully compare RR intervals. Callipers may help.

Alternatively, plot two QRS complexes on a piece of paper. Then move the paper to other sections on the rhythm strip and ascertain whether the marks are aligned exactly with other pairs of QRS complexes (regular QRS rhythm) or not (irregular QRS rhythm).

If the QRS rhythm is found to be irregular, determine whether it is totally irregular or whether there is a cyclical variation in the RR intervals (Resuscitation Council UK 2000).

A totally irregular QRS rhythm is most likely going to be atrial fibrillation, particularly if the morphology of the QRS complexes remains constant. If there is a cyclical pattern to the irregularity of the RR intervals, examine the relationship between the P waves and QRS complexes (see below). The presence of ectopics can render an otherwise regular QRS rhythm irregular. Determine whether they are atrial, junctional or ventricular.

QRS complexes

Measure the QRS width and establish whether it is normal or prolonged:

- *Normal* QRS width is < 0.12 s/3 small squares (Resuscitation Council UK 2000) – the impulse originates above the ventricles.
- *Prolonged* QRS width is 0.12 s/3 small squares or more – either the impulse originates above the ventricles but is conducted with bundle branch block (aberrant conduction) or the impulse originates in the ventricles.

Examine the QRS complexes and establish whether their morphology is constant. Look to see if ectopics or

extrasystoles are present. These can arise from the atria, AV junction and ventricles. By examining their morphology, it is usually possible to determine their origin.

If the ectopic QRS complex is narrow (< 0.12 s/3 small squares), the ectopic focus is situated above the ventricles. If it is wide, the ectopic focus is either above the ventricles, but the impulse is conducted with bundle branch block, or in the ventricles. If they are premature, i.e. before the next anticipated sinus beat, they are commonly termed premature contractions. If they are late, i.e. after the next anticipated sinus beat – e.g. following a period of sinus arrest – they are commonly termed escape beats.

P waves

Establish whether P waves are present. If they are present, determine the rate and whether their morphology is constant.

In sinus rhythm the P waves should be identical in shape and upright in lead II. Changes in P wave morphology implies a different pacemaker focus for the impulse. Retrograde activation through the AV junction (junctional or ventricular arrhythmias) usually results in the P waves being inverted in lead II. This is because atrial depolarisation occurs in the opposite direction to normal.

Sometimes it may be difficult to establish whether P waves are present because they are partly or totally obscured by the QRS complexes or T waves, e.g. in sinus tachycardia P waves may merge with the preceding T waves.

In SA block and sinus arrest, P waves will be absent. In atrial fibrillation no P waves can be identified, just a fluctuating baseline. In atrial flutter, P waves are replaced by regular sawtooth flutter waves, rate approximately 300/min.

Relationship between P waves and QRS complexes

Establish whether the P waves and QRS complexes are 'married' to each other. Ascertain whether each P wave is followed by a QRS complex and each QRS complex is preceded by a P wave.

Examine the PR interval. The normal PR interval is 0.12–0.20 s (3–5 small squares). Causes of a shortened PR interval include junctional rhythms and impulse conduction via accessory conduction pathways, e.g. bundle of Kent (Wolff–Parkinson–White syndrome). AV block can cause a prolonged PR interval.

If the PR interval is constant, atrial and ventricular activity is likely to be associated. If the PR interval is variable, establish whether atrial and ventricular activity is associated or dissociated. Map out the P waves and QRS complexes and examine their relationship. Look for any recognisable patterns, the presence of dropped beats and PR intervals that vary in a repeated fashion (Resuscitation Council UK 2000).

AV dissociation is when the atria and ventricles are depolarised by two different sources. It is seen for example in 3rd degree AV block and ventricular tachycardia. It is not a diagnosis in itself, but a clinical feature, identified on the ECG of a cardiac arrhythmia.

CHAPTER SUMMARY

Accurate ECG interpretation of cardiac arrhythmias is essential to ensure the most appropriate management. In this chapter a five-stage approach to ECG interpretation of cardiac arrhythmias has been described.

REFERENCES

Esberger, D., Jones, S. & Morris, F. (2002) ABC of clinical electrocardiography: junctional tachycardias. *British Medical Journal* **324**: 662–5.

Jowett, N.I. & Thompson, D.R. (1995) *Comprehensive Coronary Care*, 2nd edn. Scutari Press, London.

Julian, D. & Cowan, J. (1993) *Cardiology*, 6th edn. Baillière, London.

Meltzer, L.E., Pinneo, R. & Kitchell, J.R. (1983) *Intensive Coronary Care: A Manual for Nurses*, 4th edn. Prentice Hall, London.

Resuscitation Council UK (2000) *Advanced Life Support Manual*, 4th edn. Resuscitation Council UK, London.

Tonkin, A. (1997) Pathophysiology of post infarction ventricular arrhythmias, in Thompson, P. (ed.) *Coronary Care Manual*. Churchill Livingstone, London.

Cardiac Arrhythmias Originating in the SA Node

INTRODUCTION

Cardiac arrhythmias originating in the SA node result from a disturbance in impulse formation or impulse conduction within the node itself. The SA node retains its role as pacemaker for the heart, but instead of firing regularly at a rate of 60–100/min, it is firing at a slower, faster or irregular rate. Sometimes the SA node fails to discharge an impulse and activate the atria, either because the impulse is blocked within the node itself or it fails to initiate an impulse.

The aim of this chapter is to recognise cardiac arrhythmias originating in the SA node.

LEARNING OBJECTIVES

At the end of the chapter the reader will be able to discuss the characteristic ECG features, list the causes and outline the treatment of:

❏ sinus tachycardia;
❏ sinus bradycardia;
❏ sinus arrhythmia;
❏ wandering atrial pacemaker;
❏ SA block;
❏ SA arrest;
❏ sick sinus syndrome.

SINUS TACHYCARDIA

Sinus tachycardia can be defined as a sinus rhythm greater than 100 beats/min (Bennett 1994). The ECG has the same characteristics as sinus rhythm, except that the QRS rate is greater than 100 beats/min. The upper limit of sinus tachycardia is usually 140 beats/min (Jowett & Thompson 1995). Sinus tachycardia at rest is a normal finding in infancy and early childhood (Camm & Katritsis 1996).

A classical feature which helps distinguish sinus tachycardia from other narrow complex tachycardias, e.g. atrial tachycardia, is that it does not start and end abruptly; both its onset and decline are gradual (Thompson 1997). Sometimes in sinus tachycardia, P waves can merge with the preceding QRS complexes.

Sinus tachycardia can be a normal response to physiological stimuli. However, if it persists it is usually an indication of pathophysiology (Randall & Ardell 1990). Causes include anxiety, hypovolaemia, exercise, shock, pyrexia and drugs such as hydralazine, nebulised salbutamol. Of greater impor-

tance is that it may be a manifestation of heart failure when it is a reflex mechanism to compensate for reduced stroke volume (Meltzer *et al*. 1983).

In myocardial infarction, sinus tachycardia is an adverse prognostic sign (Hjalmarson *et al*. 1990), because it is usually indicates extensive myocardial necrosis associated with excess release of catecholamines (Thompson 1997). Persistent tachycardia suggests an extensive myocardial infarction (ISIS 2 1988).

Persistent tachycardia in the absence of any obvious underlying cause should prompt consideration of atrial tachyacrdia or atrial flutter (Goodacre & Irons 2002).

Identifying features on the ECG

- *QRS rate*: > 100/min, usually < 140/min.
- *QRS rhythm*: regular.
- *QRS complexes*: normal width and constant morphology.

- *P waves*: present, may be merged into preceding T waves.
- *Relationship between P waves and QRS complexes*: each P wave is followed by a QRS complex and each QRS complex is preceded by a P wave; PR interval is normal and constant.

Effects on the patient

Most patients with sinus tachycardia are asymptomatic. However, some may complain of palpitations and dyspnoea (Thompson 1997). As the rate increases the resultant decreased arterial pressure filling time and reduced stroke volume may lead to a drop in blood pressure and weak peripheral pulses.

Sinus tachycardia will increase oxygen consumption and, when associated with myocardial infarction, could extend myocardial necrosis (Jevon 2002).

Treatment

Treatment is generally aimed at identifying and, where appropriate, treating the cause. It must be stressed that the intentional slowing down of a sinus tachycardia when it is a normal compensatory mechanism, e.g. in left ventricular failure, can have disastrous consequences on the patient.

In myocardial infarction, underlying causes should be sought and appropriate treatment instigated promptly (White 1996). The use of beta-blocking agents, e.g. atenolol, can benefit some patients (ISIS 1 1986). Sometimes the tachycardia may be pain and/or anxiety induced and may settle with effective pain relief. Any electrolyte imbalances should be corrected. Rarely catheter ablation therapy on the sinus node is undertaken if drugs have failed to control the rate (Davis 1997).

Interpretation of Fig. 4.1

- *QRS rate*: 115/min.
- *QRS rhythm*: regular.
- *QRS*: normal width and constant morphology; ST elevation is present.

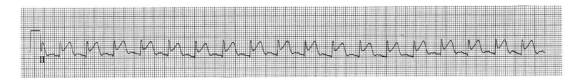

Fig. 4.1 Sinus tachycardia

- *P waves*: present, constant morphology.
- *Relationship between P waves and QRS complexes*: each P wave is followed by a QRS complex and each QRS complex is preceded by a P wave; PR interval is normal and constant.

The ECG in Fig. 4.1 displays sinus tachycardia. This patient was admitted to CCU with an acute inferior myocardial infarction (the ST elevation is suggestive of myocardial damage; a 12 lead ECG helped to confirm this diagnosis). He was complaining of severe central chest pain and was very anxious.

Sinus tachycardia, and not bradycardia, is an unusual clinical finding in an inferior myocardial infarction and it was important to try to identify the underlying cause. Possible causes included patient anxiety, chest pain, heart failure and cardiogenic shock. Following diamorphine 5 mg administered i.v., the patient's pain eased and he settled. The heart rate gradually slowed down to 65 beats/min. Chest pain and anxiety were the most probable underlying causes of the sinus tachycardia. There was no clinical evidence of a low cardiac output. The patient's blood pressure and respiratory rate were within normal limits.

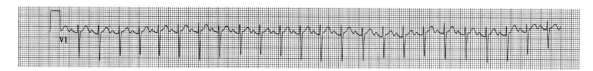

Fig. 4.2 Sinus tachycardia

Interpretation of Fig. 4.2

- *QRS rate*: 150/min.
- *QRS rhythm*: regular.
- *QRS*: normal width and constant morphology.
- *P waves*: present and constant morphology.
- *Relationship between P waves and QRS complexes*: each P wave is followed by a QRS complex and each QRS complex is preceded by a P wave; PR interval is normal and constant.

This patient was referred by his general practitioner with a sudden onset of dyspnoea. The ECG displays sinus tachycardia with a ventricular rate of 150/min.

BP was 90/60, respiratory rate was 34/min and the patient was pale, cold and clammy. He was also orthopnoec and expectorating frothy bloodstained sputum. Auscultation confirmed the presence of pulmonary oedema.

It is likely that the sinus tachycardia was secondary to acute left ventricular failure. Following effective treatment of the primary problem with oxygen, diuretics, nitrates and a small dose of diamorphine, the patient settled and the tachycardia gradually slowed (a characteristic sign of sinus tachycardia).

This is an unusually rapid rate for sinus tachycardia. A tachycardia of this rate could have been caused by an atrial tachyarrhythmia, e.g. atrial tachycardia. However, the PR interval is normal, not short. Close inspection of the 12 lead ECG did confirm sinus tachycardia.

SINUS BRADYCARDIA

Sinus bradycardia can be defined as a sinus rhythm of less than 60/min. The ECG has the same characteristics as sinus rhythm, except that the QRS rate is less than 60/min.

The commonest cause of sinus bradycardia is acute myocardial infarction (Da Costa *et al.* 2002), particularly inferior myocardial infarction (Adgey *et al.* 1971), being caused by increased parasympathetic tone (White 1996). Other causes include certain medical conditions such as hypothermia (Resuscitation Council UK 2000) and hypothyroidism (Vanhaelst & Neve 1967), vagal stimulation, e.g. during tracheal suction, increased intracranial pressure, hypoxia, severe pain, hypothermia and drugs such as beta-blockers. It can be a normal clinical finding in some patients, e.g. athletes.

Sinus bradycardia may also be caused by sinus node dysfunction (Levy & Mogensen 1996). Conditions associated with sinus node dysfunction include age, ischaemia, high vagal tone, myocarditis and digoxin toxicity (Da Costa *et al.* 2002).

Identifying features on the ECG

- *QRS rate*: < 60/min.
- *QRS rhythm*: regular.
- *QRS complexes*: normal width and constant morphology.
- *P waves*: present, constant morphology.
- *Relationship between P waves and QRS complexes*: P wave is followed by a QRS complex and each QRS complex is preceded by a P wave; PR interval is normal and constant.

Effects on the patient

Many patients are able to tolerate heart rates of 40/min surprisingly well (Da Costa *et al.* 2002). Some patients are asymptomatic. It can be a normal physiological state in fit people, e.g. athletes. It may the desired effect of beta-blocker drug administration. It is common in the early stages of inferior myocardial infarction, rarely requiring treatment (Nolan *et al.* 1998).

However, the patient may be symptomatic, particularly if the bradycardia is of a sudden onset. Symptoms (of decreased cardiac output) include hypotension, chest pain, lightheadiness, dizziness, nausea, syncope, and pale, clammy skin. In addition, escape rhythms are more likely to occur which can predispose to ventricular tachyarrhythmias (Jowett & Thompson 1995).

Treatment

Treatment is indicated only if adverse signs (see pages 189–90) are present and/or there is a risk of asystole (Resuscitation Council UK 2000). If necessary, oxygen should be administered and i.v. access secured. If treatment is required, atropine 500 mcg should be administered i.v. and the ECG rhythm reassessed. Further doses may be required. Cardiac pacing may be

required in some situations. The possible cause of the bradycardia should be established, as attention to this (e.g. omitting medication) may provide the most effective treatment. Any electrolyte imbalances should be corrected.

Interpretation of Fig. 4.3

- *QRS rate*: 42/min.
- *QRS rhythm*: regular.
- *QRS complex*: normal width and constant morphology.
- *P waves*: present and constant morphology.
- *Relationship between P waves and QRS complexes*: each P wave is followed by a QRS complex and each QRS complex is preceded by a P wave; PR interval normal and constant.

The ECG in Fig. 4.3 displays sinus bradycardia. The ECG has the same characteristics as sinus rhythm except that the QRS rate is < 60 beats/min. This patient

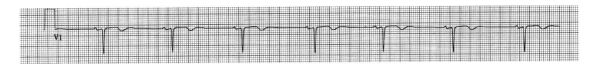

Fig. 4.3 Sinus bradycardia

had been admitted with an acute inferior myocardial infarction (the most common cause of bradycardia).

In myocardial infarction, bradycardia reduces myocardial oxygen requirements and, as long as the patient remains asymptomatic, no treatment is required (White 1996). The patient did not present with any adverse signs (see pages 189–90) and he was not taking any medications prior to admission that could cause a bradycardia (e.g. a beta-blocker). The blood pressure was stable, the bradycardia transient and no treatment was required. However, the patient was closely monitored during the period of bradycardia in order to detect the occurrence of adverse signs.

Interpretation of Fig. 4.4

- *QRS rate*: 26/min.
- *QRS rhythm*: regular.
- *QRS complex*: very wide (0.16 s or 4 small squares) and constant morphology.
- *P waves*: present and constant morphology.
- *Relationship between P waves and QRS complexes*: each P wave is followed by a QRS complex and each QRS complex is preceded by a P wave; PR interval normal and constant.

The ECG in Fig. 4.4 displays profound sinus bradycardia. The ECG has the same characteristics as sinus

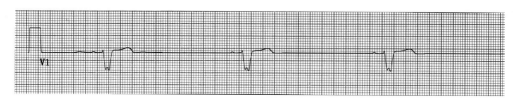

Fig. 4.4 Sinus bradycardia

rhythm except that the QRS rate is < 60 beats/min. In addition the QRS complex is very wide, suggestive of bundle branch block (a 12 lead ECG confirmed left bundle branch block).

This patient had been admitted with an acute anterior myocardial infarction. The patient was assessed for the presence of adverse signs (see pages 189–90). BP was 75/40 and the patient was semi-conscious. He was also very pale and clammy, though these signs are often associated with acute myocardial infarction.

It was quickly established that the patient was severely haemodynamically compromised and urgent intervention to treat the bradycardia was required. The patient was placed in as supine position and oxygen was administered. Atropine 500 mcg was administered i.v. and then the patient was reassessed. Despite further doses of atropine, the bradycardia did not respond and the patient remained compromised. External pacing, quickly followed by transvenous pacing, was required. This patient needed a permanent pacemaker.

SINUS ARRHYTHMIA

Sinus arrhythmia is a variation of sinus rhythm characterised by alternate periods of slow and more rapid sinus node discharge (Reynolds 1996). The ECG characteristics are the same except that the QRS rhythm is slightly irregular. It is a normal finding and is usually associated with the phases of respiration, increasing with inspiration and decreasing with expiration.

Sometimes sinus arrhythmia is associated with ischaemia or digoxin toxicity (Reynolds 1996). In addition, the irregular QRS rhythm can be mistaken for other arrhythmias, e.g. atrial fibrillation.

Identifying features on the ECG

- *QRS rate*: 60–100/min.
- *QRS rhythm*: slightly irregular.
- *QRS width*: normal and constant morphology.
- *P waves*: present and constant morphology.
- *Relationship between P waves and QRS complexes*: each P wave is followed by a QRS complex and each QRS complex is preceded by a P wave; PR interval normal and constant.

Effects on the patient

No ill effects reported.

Treatment

No treatment required. Any electrolyte imbalances should be corrected.

Interpretation of Fig. 4.5

- *QRS rate*: 75/min.
- *QRS rhythm*: slightly irregular.
- *QRS width*: normal and constant morphology.
- *P waves*: present and constant morphology.
- *Relationship between P waves and QRS complexes*: each P wave is followed by a QRS complex and each QRS complex is preceded by a P wave; PR interval normal and constant.

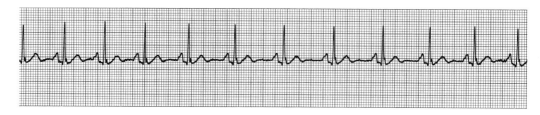

Fig. 4.5 Sinus arrhythmia

The ECG in Fig. 4.5 displays sinus arrhythmia. Close inspection confirmed the irregularity of the rhythm was not a serious arrhythmia, e.g. atrial fibrillation. This ECG strip was recorded in a 37-year-old male. The heart rate fluctuated with respiration.

WANDERING ATRIAL PACEMAKER

A wandering atrial pacemaker is characterised by the pacemaker 'wandering' from the SA node down to the atria or AV junction. It is usually related to vagal influ-ences (Meltzer *et al*. 1983). It can occur in healthy young people, but it may be a manifestation of atrial pathology (Thompson 1997).

Identifying features on the ECG

- *QRS rate*: usually normal.
- *QRS rhythm*: regular.
- *QRS complexes*: normal width and constant morphology.

- *P waves*: present, morphology and position will vary depending on the site of origin of the impulse.
- *Relationship between P waves and QRS complexes*: each P wave is followed by a QRS complex and each QRS complex is preceded by a P wave; PR interval may vary depending on the site of the origin of the impulse.

Effects on the patient

The are no effects on the patient.

Treatment

No treatment required. Any electrolyte imbalances should be corrected.

SA BLOCK

In SA block the impulse from the node itself is blocked and fails to transverse the junction between the SA node and the surrounding atrial myocardium (Bennett 1994). This results in a dropped beat. Just as with AV junctional block, SA block can be classified as 1st, 2nd and 3rd degree block.

However, only 2nd degree SA block can be diagnosed from the ECG. Intermittent failure of atrial activation results in PP intervals which are multiples (usually twice) of the cycle length during sinus rhythm (Bennett 1994). On the ECG a complete PQRST complex is absent, but the next sinus beat arises at the expected time.

Causes of SA block include idiopathic fibrosis of the SA node, cardiomyopathy, myocardial ischaemia/ infarction.

Identifying features on the ECG

- *QRS rate*: usually normal, sometimes < 60/min.
- *QRS rhythm*: dropped beats results in an irregular rhythm.
- *QRS complexes*: normal width and constant morphology.

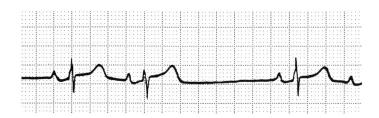

Fig. 4.6 SA block

- *P waves*: absent during period of SA block, otherwise present and constant morphology.
- *Relationship between P waves and QRS complexes*: PQRST complex absent during period of SA block, otherwise each P wave is followed by a QRS complex and each QRS complex is preceded by a P wave; PR interval normal and constant.

Effects on the patient

Rarely affects the patient, although syncope may occur if pauses are prolonged or occur frequently.

Treatment

SA block is of little clinical importance, except that it may be a manifestation of intoxication by digoxin or other anti-arrhythmic drugs (Julian & Cowan 1993). Dose reduction or withdrawal of drug(s) that the patient is taking may be required. Any electrolyte imbalances should be corrected.

Interpretation of Fig. 4.6

- *QRS rate*: approximately 60–70/min.
- *QRS rhythm*: dropped beats results in an irregular rhythm.

- *QRS complexes*: normal width and constant morphology, one dropped beat.
- *P waves*: absent during period of SA block, otherwise present and constant morphology; PP intervals are constant despite the dropped beat – this is suggestive of SA block.
- *Relationship between P waves and QRS complexes*: PQRST complex absent during period of SA block, otherwise each P wave is followed by a QRS complex and each QRS complex is preceded by a P wave; PR interval normal and constant.

The ECG in Fig. 4.6 displays 2nd degree SA block. The patient did not display any adverse signs and there were no episodes of syncope. The patient had been taking digoxin (125 mcg once daily) for several years for 'atrial fibrillation'. As the ECG trace displays, the patient was no longer in atrial fibrillation, and because the arrhythmia could have been caused by digoxin, the drug was stopped while the patient's digoxin levels were measured.

SINUS ARREST

Sinus arrest is when the SA node fails to initiate an impulse. It is characterised by absent P waves and cardiac standstill for varying periods of time, with escape beats from the atria, AV junction or ventricles taking over (hopefully) pacemaker function (escape rhythm) (Jowett & Thompson 1995).

Causes of sinus arrest include idiopathic fibrosis of the SA node, cardiomyopathy and myocardial ischaemia/infarction. Intermittent sinus arrest may occur following an inferior myocardial infarction or as a vagal efferent response to the Bezold–Jarisch reflex during right coronary artery reperfusion (Koren *et al*. 1986).

Identifying features on the ECG

- *QRS rate*: normal or < 60/min.
- *QRS rhythm*: irregular due to dropped beats.
- *QRS complexes*: usually normal width and constant morphology; if escape beats present these may be of

different morphology depending on their site of origin.

- *P waves*: absent during period of SA block, otherwise present and constant morphology.
- *Relationship between P waves and QRS complexes*: PQRST complex absent during period of sinus arrest, otherwise each P wave is followed by a QRS complex and each QRS complex is preceded by a P wave; PR interval normal and constant.

Effects on the patient

Although the haemodynamic effect on the patient is usually self-limiting owing to the junctional or ventricular escape beats maintaining a cardiac output, it may still be severe enough to cause syncope (Thompson 1997).

Treatment

Atropine will be required during periods of sinus arrest if adverse signs (see pages 189–90) are present (Nolan *et al*. 1998). If recurrent and causing syncope, a permanent pacemaker may be required (Thompson 1997). Any electrolyte imbalances should be corrected.

Interpretation of Fig. 4.7

- *QRS rate*: difficult to determine (longer ECG strip required).
- *QRS rhythm*: irregular, 4.5 s pause present.
- *QRS complexes*: normal width and constant morphology.
- *P waves*: absent during sinus arrest, otherwise present and constant morphology.
- *Relationship between P waves and QRS complexes*: absent QRS complexes owing to sinus arrest and no escape rhythms present; otherwise each P wave is followed by a QRS complex and each QRS complex is preceded by a P wave; PR interval normal and constant.

The ECG in Fig. 4.7 displays sinus arrest. Profound adverse signs were present. BP was unrecordable and the patient was cold, pale, clammy, semi-conscious and agitated.

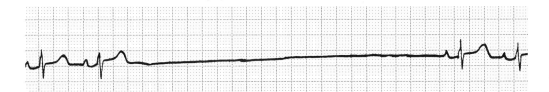

Fig. 4.7 Sinus arrest

It was quickly established that the patient was severely haemodynamically compromised and urgent intervention to treat the sinus arrest and the resultant bradycardia was required. The patient was placed in a supine position and oxygen administered. Atropine 500 mcg was administered i.v. and the patient reassessed. After a second dose of atropine, the heart rate did improve. The sinus arrest was transient and the cause was thought to be inferior myocardial ischaemia. No further treatment was required.

SICK SINUS SYNDROME

Sick sinus syndrome is the term used to describe a condition that encompasses a variety of cardiac arrhythmias related to abnormal SA node and atrial activity (Ferrer 1973). A common cause of syncope, dizzy episodes and palpitations, sick sinus syndrome is more common in the elderly although it may occur at any age (Bennett 1994).

Sick sinus syndrome can be classified as follows:

- intermittent sinus arrest;
- stable sinus bradycardia;
- tachycardia–bradycardia ('tachy–brady') syndrome
  – the tachycardia is usually atrial fibrillation.

Thompson 1997

The exact cause of sick sinus syndrome is unknown, although histologic degeneration of the SA node, AV junction and the conduction tissues between the two is often found on post-mortem (Ornato & Peberdy 1996).

Identifying features on the ECG
Identifying features will depend on the arrhythmias (see above).

Effects on the patient
The patient may complain of palpitations if tachy-arrhythmic episodes present. During periods of severe bradycardia or asystole the patient may experience a syncope attack.

Treatment
Patients with persistent symptomatic bradycardia usually require permanent ventricular or AV sequential pacing (Ornato & Peberdy 1996). Patients with the tachy–brady syndrome may also require concurrent anti-arrhythmic therapy. However, with the increasing use of DDD chamber pacemakers, sick sinus syndrome can often be controlled with just pacemaker therapy (Thompson 1997). Any electrolyte imbalances should be corrected.

CHAPTER SUMMARY
Cardiac arrhythmias originating in the SA node result from a disturbance in impulse formation or impulse conduction within the node itself. The SA node usually retains its role as pacemaker for the heart, but instead of firing regularly at a rate of 60–100/min, it is firing at a slower (sinus bradycardia), faster (sinus tachycardia) or irregular (sinus arrhythmia) rate. Sometimes the SA node fails to discharge an impulse and activate the atria, either because the impulse is blocked (SA

block) within the node itself or because it fails to initiate an impulse (sinus arrest).

REFERENCES

Adgey, A., Geddes, J., Webb, S. *et al.* (1971) Acute phase of myocardial infarction. *Lancet* **2**: 501–4.

Bennett, D.H. (1994) *Cardiac Arrhythmias*, 4th edn. Butterworth Heinemann, Oxford.

Camm, A. & Katritsis, D. (1996) The diagnosis of tachyarrhythmias, in Julian, D. *et al.* (eds) *Diseases of the Heart*, 2nd edn. W.B. Saunders, London.

Da Costa, D., Brady, W. & Redhouse, J. (2002) ABC of clinical electrocardiography: bradycardias and atrioventricular block. *British Medical Journal* **324**: 535–8.

Davis, M. (1997) Catheter ablation therapy of arrhythmias, in Thompson, P. (ed.) *Coronary Care Manual*. Churchill Livingstone, London.

Ferrer, M. (1973) The sick sinus syndrome. *Circulation* **47**: 635–41.

Goodacre, S. & Irons, R. (2002) ABC of clinical electrocardiography: atrial arrythmias. *British Medical Journal* **324**: 594–7.

Hjalmarson, A., Gilpin, E., Kjekshus, J. *et al.* (1990) Influence of heart rate on mortality after myocardial infarction. *American Journal of Cardiology* **65**: 547–53.

ISIS 1 (First International Study of Infarct Survival) (1986) Collaborative Group. A randomised trail of intravenous atenolol among 16 027 cases of suspected myocardial infarction. *Lancet* **2**: 57–66.

ISIS 2 (1988) Collaborative group randomised trial of intravenous streptokinase, oral aspirin, both, or neither among 17 187 cases of suspected acute myocardial infarction. *Lancet* **2**: 349.

Jevon, P. (2002) *Advanced Cardiac Life Support*. Butterworth Heinemann, Oxford.

Jowett, N.I. & Thompson, D.R. (1995) *Comprehensive Coronary Care*, 2nd edn. Scutari Press, London.

Julian, D. & Cowan, J. (1993) *Cardiology*, 6th edn. Baillière, London.

Koren, G., Weiss, A., Ben-David, Y. *et al.* (1986) Bradycardia and hypotension following reperfusion with streptokinase (Bezold–Jarisch reflex): a sign of coronary thrombolysis and myocardial salvage. *American Heart Journal* **112**: 468–71.

Levy, S. & Mogensen, L. (1996) Diagnosis of bradycardias, in Julian, D. *et al.* (eds) *Diseases of the Heart*, 2nd edn. W.B. Saunders, London.

Meltzer, L.E., Pinneo, R. & Kitchell, J.R. (1983) *Intensive Coronary Care: A Manual for Nurses*, 4th edn. Prentice Hall, London.

Nolan. J., Greenwood, J. & Mackintosh, A. (1998) *Cardiac*

Emergencies: A Pocket Guide. Butterworth Heinemann, Oxford.

Ornato, J. & Peberdy, M. (1996) Etiology, electrophysiology, and myocardial mechanics of bradyasystolic states, in Paradis, N., Halperin, H. & Nowak, R. (eds) *Cardiac Arrest: The Science and Practice of Resuscitation Medicine*. Williams & Wilkins, London.

Randall, W. & Ardell, J. (1990) Nervous control of the heart: anatomy and pathophysiology, in Zipes, D. & Jalife, J. (eds) *Cardiac Electrophysiology: From Cell to Bedside*. W.B. Saunders, Philadelphia.

Resuscitation Council UK (2000) *Advanced Life Support Manual*, 4th edn. Resuscitation Council UK, London.

Reynolds, G. (1996) The resting electrocardiogram, in Julian, D. *et al*. (eds) *Diseases of the Heart*, 2nd edn. W.B. Saunders, London.

Thompson, P. (1997) *Coronary Care Manual*. Churchill Livingstone, London.

Vanhaelst, I. & Neve, P. (1967) Coronary artery disease and hypothyroidism. *Lancet* **2**: 800.

White, H. (1996) Myocardial infarction, in Julian, D. *et al*. (eds) *Diseases of the Heart*, 2nd edn. W.B. Saunders, London.

Cardiac Arrhythmias Originating in the Atria

INTRODUCTION

Cardiac arrhythmias originating in the atria result primarily from either ischaemic damage to, or overdistension of, the atrial walls. If P waves are present they are usually of different morphology from sinus P waves. As the ventricles are activated via the normal conduction pathways, the QRS complex is usually narrow and of a normal morphology.

Any complications resulting from atrial arrhythmias are usually associated with the tachycardic rate and/or loss of effective atrial contractions (atrial kick).

The aim of this chapter is to recognise cardiac arrhythmias originating in the atria.

LEARNING OBJECTIVES

At the end of the chapter the reader will be able to discuss the characteristic ECG features, list the causes and outline the treatment of:

❏ atrial premature beats;
❏ atrial tachycardia;
❏ atrial flutter;
❏ atrial fibrillation.

ATRIAL PREMATURE BEATS

Atrial premature beats (APBs) are caused by an ectopic focus in the atria (and very occasionally in the SA node itself) (Camm & Katritsis 1996). They can be a normal finding and can be worsened by cardiac stimulants, e.g. tobacco, caffeine and alcohol (Thompson 1997). They can complicate heart disease, especially atrial enlargement, and may herald the onset of atrial fibrillation, atrial flutter or atrial tachycardia.

APBs occur prior to the next anticipated sinus beat (Camm & Katritsis 1996). They have abnormally shaped P waves, normal QRS complexes and an ensuing pause that is approximately equal to or marginally longer than the normal sinus RR interval. Atrial bigeminy is when an APB occurs every second beat and atrial trigeminy is when an APB occurs every third beat (Marriott 1988).

Sometimes an APB is not conducted to the ventricles because it has arisen so early in the cardiac cycle that the AV junction is still refractory and unable to conduct it (see Fig. 5.3, page 61). This is a common cause of unexpected pauses (Camm & Katritsis 1996).

Identifying features on the ECG

- *QRS rate*: usually normal, though dependent upon underlying rhythm and frequency of APBs.

- *QRS rhythm*: slightly irregular owing to presence of APBs.
- *QRS complexes*: usually normal width and constant morphology; the prematurity of the APB may result in the impulse being conducted to the ventricles with bundle branch block – QRS morphology will then differ.
- *P waves*: present; those associated with APBs will be of different morphology from sinus P waves and may be superimposed on the preceding T waves.
- *Relationship between P waves and QRS complexes*: each P wave is followed by a QRS complex and each QRS complex is preceded by a P wave; PR interval may be marginally longer than in sinus rhythm (Camm & Katritsis 1996).

Effects on the patient

The most common symptom is palpitations; the patient is usually aware of the premature contraction itself, of the following pause often described as a 'missed beat' or of a stronger post-ectopic beat (Camm

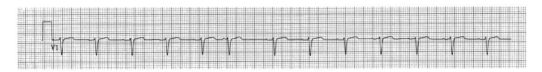

Fig. 5.1 Atrial premature beat

& Katritsis 1996). The palpitations are more evident at night when the patient is in a left lateral position, during or immediately following exercise and while sitting quietly (Camm & Katritsis 1996). On rare occasions the patient may experience chest pain. The patient may be asymptomatic.

Treatment

APBs are benign and no treatment is necessary. Any electrolyte imbalances should be corrected.

Interpretation of Fig. 5.1

- *QRS rate*: 75/min.
- *QRS rhythm*: slightly irregular owing to APB.

- *QRS complexes*: normal width and constant morphology.
- *P waves*: present; the P wave associated with the APB is of different morphology from the sinus P waves.
- *Relationship between P waves and QRS complexes*: each P wave is followed by a QRS complex and each QRS complex is preceded by a P wave; the PR interval associated with the APB is shorter than the PR interval in the sinus beats.

The ECG in Fig. 5.1 displays sinus rhythm with an APB. This patient was admitted to the ward with increasing episodes of angina. When checking her pulse, it was found to be slightly irregular. Cardiac

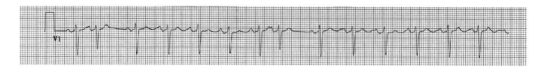

Fig. 5.2 Frequent atrial premature beats

monitoring confirmed that this was due to the presence of occasional APBs. No treatment was required. In fact, a few hours after admission the APBs ceased occurring, thus suggesting their likely underlying cause to be patient anxiety.

Interpretation of Fig. 5.2

- *QRS rate*: 95/min.
- *QRS rhythm*: slightly irregular owing to presence of APBs.
- *QRS complexes*: normal width and constant morphology.

- *P waves*: present, those associated with the APBs are superimposed on the preceding T waves – not possible to assess their morphology.
- *Relationship between P waves and QRS complexes*: each P wave is followed by a QRS complex and each QRS complex is preceded by a P wave; PR interval associated with the APBs is difficult to calculate.

The ECG in Fig. 5.2 displays sinus rhythm with APBs. This patient was admitted to the ward with a history of palpitations and thyrotoxicosis. There were no adverse signs present. However, the patient was commenced on cardiac monitoring because the

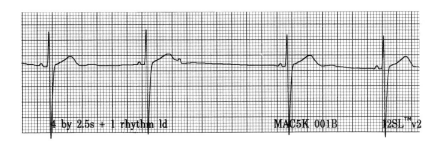

Fig. 5.3 Non-conducted atrial premature beat

frequency of APBs together with a diagnosis of thyrotoxicosis increased the probability of atrial arrhythmias, particularly atrial fibrillation.

Interpretation of Fig. 5.3

- *QRS rate*: approximately 50/min.
- *QRS rhythm*: slightly irregular owing to presence of APB.
- *QRS complexes*: normal width and constant morphology.

- *P waves*: present; one (APB) has occurred very early in the cardiac cycle.
- *Relationship between P waves and QRS complexes*: except for one P wave (APB), each P wave is followed by a QRS complex and each QRS complex is preceded by a P wave; PR interval constant.

The ECG in Fig. 5.3 displays a non-conducted APB, resulting in a pause. The APB has not been conducted to the ventricles because it has arisen so early in the cycle that the AV junction is still refractory and unable to conduct it. This was only an isolated non-conducted APB and no treatment was required.

ATRIAL TACHYCARDIA

Atrial tachycardia is caused by an ectopic focus in the atria. It is often preceded by premature atrial contractions and is characterised by a sudden onset and an abrupt end (Meltzer *et al.* 1983). The atrial rate is normally between 150 and 250/min (Goodacre & Irons 2002). Although the AV junction may conduct all the impulses, there is often a degree of AV block (Bennett 1994), particularly if there is associated digoxin toxicity. Other causes of artial tachycardia include cardiomyopathy, sick sinus syndrome, ischaemic heart disease and rheumatic heart disease.

Multifocal atrial tachycardia can occur in critically ill elderly patients with respiratory disease. It is characterised by multiple atrial foci resulting in P waves of varying morphology and of a variable rate (Nolan *et al.* 1998).

Carotid sinus massage is often helpful with diagnosis (Bennett 1994). It produces a transient increase in AV block with a corresponding drop in the ventricular rate (Julian & Cowan 1993). Adenosine may also aid diagnosis (Goodacre & Irons 2002).

Identifying features on the ECG

- *QRS rate*: usually 150–200/min.
- *QRS rhythm*: regular.
- *QRS complexes*: normal width and morphology.
- *P waves*: rate between 150 and 250/min, may not be visible, may be merged into preceding T waves; if visible, different morphology from sinus P waves.
- *Relationship between P waves and QRS complexes*: difficult to ascertain relationship; PR interval often cannot be determined because P waves are not clearly distinguishable; if there is AV block, P waves may not be conducted to the ventricles (usually 2:1 AV block, i.e. every other P wave is blocked).

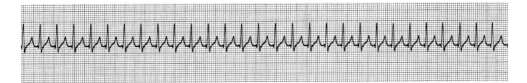

Fig. 5.4 Atrial tachycardia

Effects on the patient

Atrial tachycardia may be associated with palpitations or haemodynamic compromise due to the loss of effective atrial contractions and a rapid ventricular rate.

Treatment

Vagal manoeuvres and adenosine may be effective at terminating the arrhythmia. If the patient is taking digoxin, toxicity should be suspected and the digoxin should be omitted (Bennett 1994). Cardioversion should be avoided in these patients because it may produce intractable arrhythmias (Nolan *et al.* 1998). Any electrolyte imbalances should be corrected.

The treatment of multifocal atrial tachycardia associated with respiratory disease is to ensure that serum potassium levels are adequate and to treat the underlying respiratory problem (Nolan *et al.* 1998).

Interpretation of Fig. 5.4

- *QRS rate*: 180/min.
- *QRS rhythm*: regular.

- *QRS complexes*: normal width and constant morphology.
- *P waves*: present on the preceding T waves.
- *Relationship between P waves and QRS complexes*: each P wave is followed by a QRS complex and each QRS complex is preceded by a P wave; PR interval constant.

The ECG in Fig. 5.4 displays atrial tachycardia. The patient was admitted to the coronary ward with palpitations. There were no adverse signs present. His blood pressure was stable and there were no signs of reduced cardiac output (see pages 189–90). Carotid sinus massage applied by the doctor was ineffective. Adenosine 6 mg was then administered i.v., but without success. Three further doses of 12 mg each were also unsuccessful. As there were no adverse signs present (i.e. patient did not require cardioversion at that stage), amiodarone 300 mg was administered i.v. over 1 hour. This was successful at terminating the arrhythmia. The patient's haemodynamic status was monitored throughout in order to promptly detect the presence of adverse signs, i.e. the patient was becoming unstable.

ATRIAL FLUTTER

Atrial flutter is less common than atrial fibrillation and is nearly always associated with significant cardiac disease, e.g. mitral valve disease (Nolan *et al.* 1998). It complicates 2–5% of acute myocardial infarctions (Marriott & Meyerburg 1986).

It is characterised by a zigzagging baseline which produces the typical sawtooth flutter (F) waves, often most evident in the inferior leads and in lead V1 (Goodacre & Irons 2002). If this characteristic pattern is not initially obvious, it can be frequently visualised by applying carotid sinus massage to increase AV block (Thompson 1997).

Atrial flutter is often initiated by an atrial premature beat and may degenerate into atrial fibrillation (Bennett 1994). In the majority of cases the atrial rate is 300/min and only alternate F waves are conducted to the ventricles (2:1 AV block) (Camm & Katritsis 1996). The presence of a regular tachycardia with this rate should prompt the possible diagnosis of atrial flutter (Goodacre & Irons 2002).

Identifying features on the ECG

- *QRS rate*: dependent on the degree of AV block; usually 150/min.
- *QRS rhythm*: regular or irregular (dependent on AV block).
- *QRS complexes*: normal width and constant morphology.
- *P waves*: sawtooth flutter waves present, usually 300/min; best seen in inferior leads.
- *Relationship between P waves and QRS complexes*: usually a degree of AV block is present, e.g. 2:1, 3:1 and 4:1 AV block; AV block may be variable.

Effects on the patient

Patients with atrial flutter usually present with rapid palpitations (Camm & Katritsis 1996). Sometimes atrial flutter is associated with haemodynamic compromise owing to the loss of effective atrial contractions and a rapid ventricular rate (Nolan *et al*. 1998).

Treatment

Atrial flutter usually responds to carotid sinus massage, most commonly with a decrease in ventricular rate (rarely atrial fibrillation or sinus rhythm) (Camm & Katritsis 1996).

Although class 1 anti-arrhythmic drugs, e.g. sotolol, flecainide and disopyramide, may terminate atrial flutter, if unsuccessful they may actually lead to higher ventricular rates (Bennett 1994). Amiodarone is often effective (Nolan *et al*. 1998) and synchronised cardioversion is very effective (De Silva *et al*. 1980). Overdrive atrial pacing can restore sinus rhythm in 70% of patients (Nolan *et al*. 1998). Catheter ablation has also been shown to be effective (Saoudi *et al*. 1990). Any electrolyte imbalances should be corrected.

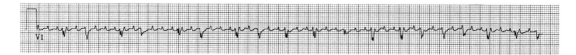

Fig. 5.5 Atrial flutter

Interpretation of Fig. 5.5

- *QRS rate*: 110/min.
- *QRS rhythm*: irregular owing to varying AV block.
- *QRS complexes*: normal width and constant morphology.
- *P waves*: flutter waves present 300/min.
- *Relationship between P waves and QRS complexes*: not every flutter wave is followed by a QRS complex but every QRS complex is preceded by a flutter wave; varying degrees of AV block present.

The ECG in Fig. 5.5 displays atrial flutter with varying degrees of AV block. This patient was haemo- dynamically stable and there were no adverse signs. Unfortunately, amiodarone was ineffective at terminating the arrhythmia. However, following synchronised cardioversion at 100 J, sinus rhythm did ensue.

Interpretation of Fig. 5.6

- *QRS rate*: 90/min.
- *QRS rhythm*: regular.
- *QRS complexes*: normal width and constant morphology.
- *P waves*: flutter waves present, rate 270/min.
- *Relationship between P waves and QRS complexes*: not

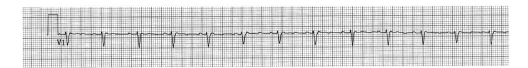

Fig. 5.6 Atrial flutter

every flutter wave is followed by a QRS complex but every QRS complex is preceded by a flutter wave; 3:1 AV block present.

The ECG in Fig. 5.6 displays atrial flutter with 3:1 AV block. This patient was not haemodynamically compromised. There were no adverse signs and BP was stable. Amiodarone 300 mg was administered i.v. over 1 hour which was effective at terminating the arrhythmia.

ATRIAL FIBRILLATION

Atrial fibrillation is characterised by completely disorganised atrial depolarisation and ineffective atrial contraction (Camm & Katritsis 1996). It is usually triggered by an APB (Zipes 1992), though it may result from a degeneration of other supraventricular tachycardias, particularly atrial tachyacrdia and flutter (Goodacre & Irons 2002). It may be paroxysmal, persistent or permanent (Goodacre & Irons 2002).

The prevalence of atrial fibrillation increases with age and is present in over 10% of patients over 75 years of age (Lake & Thompson 1991). It develops in 10–15% of patients suffering a myocardial infarction (particular extensive anterior) (Liberthson et al. 1976) and is a poor prognostic indicator (Goldberg et al. 1990). Other causes of atrial fibrillation include mitral valve disease, thyrotoxicosis and hypertensive cardiac disease.

The atria discharge at a rate of 350–600/min (Bennett 1994). These impulses bombard the AV junction and are intermittently conducted to the ventricles. This results in the characteristic totally irregular QRS rhythm. Sometimes it may be difficult to distinguish fast atrial fibrillation from other tachycardias. However, the RR interval will be irregular and the overall ventricular rate often fluctuates (Goodacre & Irons 2002). The ventricular rate will depend on the degree of AV conduction; with normal conduction the rate will be 100–180/min. Slower ventricular rates suggest a higher degree of AV block or the patient may be taking medication, e.g. digoxin (Goodacre & Irons 2002).

Identifying features on the ECG

- *QRS rate*: may be slow, normal or rapid.
- *QRS rhythm*: totally irregular (regular if third degree AV block present).
- *QRS complexes*: usually normal width and constant morphology.

- *P waves*: not present; irregular baseline owing to fibrillation waves.
- *Relationship between P waves and QRS complexes*: not applicable (no P waves present).

Effects on the patient

The loss of 'atrial kick' (atrial contraction), together with a rapid ventricular response, can lead to a fall in cardiac output of up to 50% (Nolan *et al*. 1998). Heart failure may occur, particularly if the patient has coexistent valvular heart disease or impaired left ventricular function (Nolan *et al*. 1998). A significant apex-pulse deficit may exist when the ventricular rate is rapid (Jevon 2000).

If atrial fibrillation persists for more than 48 hours, there is stasis of blood in the fibrillating atria which can lead to clot formation (Nolan *et al*. 1998). This results in an increased risk of systemic thromboembolism (Wolf *et al*. 1991). In long-term atrial fibrillation, warfarin is often administered prophylactically against embolisation (BNF 43 2002).

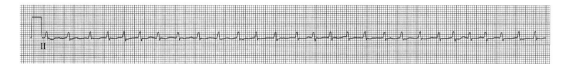

Fig. 5.7 Atrial fibrillation

Treatment

Treatment should take into account the clinical setting in which atrial fibrillation occurs; any remediable factors should be addressed if possible. The treatment is aimed at:

- slowing down the ventricular response;
- converting it to sinus rhythm (if possible);
- reducing the frequency and haemodynamic effects of subsequent atrial fibrillation or preventing further episodes.

The European Resuscitation Council guidelines for the treatment of atrial fibrillation are outlined on pages 193, 195–6. Any electrolyte imbalances should be corrected.

Interpretation of Fig. 5.7

- *QRS rate*: 160/min.
- *QRS rhythm*: irregular.
- *QRS complexes*: normal width and constant morphology.
- *P waves*: none present.
- *Relationship between P waves and QRS complexes*: not applicable (P waves not present).

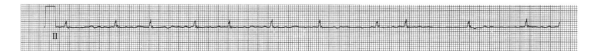

Fig. 5.8 Atrial fibrillation

The ECG in Fig. 5.7 displays atrial fibrillation with a rapid ventricular response. This patient developed atrial fibrillation as a complication of myocardial infarction. On assessment, the patient was pale, clammy, dyspnoeic and agitated; BP was 80/55. These adverse signs of poor cardiac output indicated that the patient was haemodynamically compromised and that the atrial fibrillation required urgent treatment. Following heparinisation, synchronised cardioversion 100 J was undertaken following European Resuscitation Council Guidelines (Latorre *et al.* 2001). The first shock was successful and the ECG returned to a sinus rhythm. In an attempt to prevent a recurrence of the arrhythmia, amiodarone was administered.

Interpretation of Fig. 5.8

- *QRS rate*: 70/min.
- *QRS rhythm*: irregular.
- *QRS complexes*: normal width and constant morphology.
- *P waves*: none present.
- *Relationship between P waves and QRS complexes*: not applicable (P waves not present).

The ECG in Fig. 5.8 displays atrial fibrillation. A routine 12 lead ECG prior to theatre identified this problem. There were no adverse signs and no treatment was required.

CHAPTER SUMMARY

Cardiac arrhythmias originating in the atria are generally caused by either ischaemic damage to, or overdistension of, the atrial walls. If present, P waves are of different morphology from sinus P waves. As the ventricles are activated via the normal conduction pathways, the QRS complex is usually narrow and of a normal morphology. The recognition of APBs, atrial tachycardia, atrial flutter and atrial fibrillation has been described in this chapter.

REFERENCES

BNF 43 (2002) *British National Formulary*. British Medical Association & Royal Pharmaceutical Society of Great Britain, London.

Bennett, D.H. (1994) *Cardiac Arrhythmias*, 4th edn. Butterworth Heinemann, Oxford.

Camm, A. & Katritsis, D. (1996) The diagnosis of tachyarrhythmias, in Julian, D. *et al.* (eds) *Diseases of the Heart*, 2nd edn. W.B. Saunders, London.

De Silva, R., Graboys, T., Podrid, P. & Lown, B. (1980) Cardioversion and defibrillation. *American Heart Journal* **100**: 881–95.

Goldberg, R., Seely, D., Becker, R. *et al.* (1990) Impact of atrial fibrillation on the in-hospital and long-term survival of patients with acute myocardial infarction: a community-wide perspective. *American Heart Journal* **119**: 996–1001.

Goodacre, S. & Irons, R. (2002) ABC of clinical electrocardiography: atrial arrhythmias. *British Medical Journal* **324**: 594–7.

Jevon, P. (2000) Cardiac monitoring. *Nursing Times* **96**(23): 43–4.

Julian, D. & Cowan, J. (1993) *Cardiology*, 6th edn. Baillière, London.

Lake, F. & Thompson, P. (1991) Prevention of embolic complications in non-valvular atrial fibrillation in the elderly. *Drugs and Aging* **1**(6): 458–66.

Latorre, F., Nolan, J., Robetson, C. *et al.* (2001) European Resuscitation Council Guidelines 2000 for adult advanced life support. *Resuscitation* **48**: 211–21.

Liberthson, R., Salisbury, K., Hutter, A. & De Sanctis, R. (1976) Atrial tachyarrhythmias in acute myocardial infarction. *American Journal of Medicine* **60**: 956–60.

Marriott, H. & Meyerburg, R. (1986) Recognition of arrhythmias and conduction abnormalities, in Hurst, J. (ed.) *The Heart, Arteries and Veins*. McGraw-Hill, New York.

Marriott, H.J.L. (1988) *Practical Electrocardiography*, 8th edn. Williams & Wilkins, London.

Meltzer, L.E., Pinneo, R. & Kitchell, J.R. (1983) *Intensive Coronary Care: A Manual for Nurses*, 4th edn. Prentice Hall, London.

Nolan, J., Greenwood, J. & Mackintosh, A. (1998) *Cardiac Emergencies: A Pocket Guide*. Butterworth Heinemann, Oxford.

Saoudi, N., Attalah, G., Kirkorian, G. & Touboul, P. (1990) Catheter ablation of the atrial myocardium in human type 1 atrial flutter. *Circulation* **81**: 762–71.

Thompson, P. (1997) *Coronary Care Manual*. Churchill Livingstone, London.

Wolf, P., Abbot, R. & Kannel, W. (1991) Atrial fibrillation as an independent risk factor for stroke: the Framlington Study. *Stroke* **22**: 983–8.

Zipes, D. (1992) Genesis of cardiac arrhythmias: electrophysiological considerations, in Braunwald, E. (ed.) *Heart Disease: A Textbook of Cardiovascular Medicine*, 4th edn. W.B. Saunders, Philadelphia.

Cardiac Arrhythmias Originating in the AV Junction 6

INTRODUCTION

Cardiac arrhythmias originating in the AV junction can be caused by suppression of the SA node, increased automaticity, re-entry mechanisms or blocking of the impulses in the AV junction itself. The inherent pacing rate of the AV junction is 40–60 beats/min. During junctional arrhythmias the loss of atrial kick can result in a fall in cardiac output of 20–30% (Guyton 1992).

AV re-entrant tachycardia occurs as a result of an anatomically distinct AV connection (e.g. bundle of Kent in Wolff–Parkinson–White syndrome), which permits the atrial impulse to bypass the AV node and junction and depolarise the ventricles early (ventricular pre-excitation) (Esberger *et al.* 2002).

The aim of this chapter is to recognise cardiac arrhythmias originating in the AV junction.

LEARNING OBJECTIVES

At the end of the chapter the reader will be able to discuss the characteristic ECG features, list the causes and outline the treatment of:

❏ junctional premature beats;
❏ junctional escape beats;
❏ junctional escape rhythm;

❏ junctional tachycardia;
❏ Wolff–Parkinson–White syndrome.

JUNCTIONAL PREMATURE BEATS

Junctional premature beats are less common than atrial and ventricular premature beats (Bennett 1994). They can be a normal finding and can be worsened by cardiac stimulants, e.g. tobacco, caffeine and alcohol (Thompson 1997).

Junctional premature beats are characterised by premature QRS complexes, which are of the same morphology as those associated with sinus beats. The impulses are conducted retrogradely to the atria and antegradely to the ventricles. Consequently the P waves are negative in the inferior leads and positive in aVR. The timing of the P waves in relation to the QRS complexes will depend upon the exact origin of the impulse in the AV junction: they may occur immediately before, during or following the QRS complexes (Camm & Katritsis 1996).

Identifying features on the ECG

- *QRS rate*: determined by the underlying rhythm.
- *QRS rhythm*: slightly irregular owing to junctional premature beats.
- *QRS complexes*: usually normal width and same morphology as the QRS complexes associated with sinus beats; however, the prematurity of the beat may result in the impulse being conducted to the ventricles with bundle branch block; junctional premature beats occur before the next anticipated sinus beat.
- *P waves*: usually absent; if present they will be of different morphology from those associated with sinus beats, will usually be of opposite polarity to the QRS complexes (upright in V1 or inverted in lead II) and will be located immediately prior to or following the QRS complex.
- *Relationship between P waves and QRS complexes*: if P waves present they occur immediately prior to or following the QRS complexes; if measurable, PR interval is short.

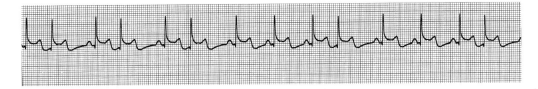

Fig. 6.1 Junctional premature beats

Effects on the patient

The patient is usually aware of a junctional premature beat, of the subsequent pause often described as a 'missed beat' or of a stronger post-ectopic beat (Camm & Katritsis 1996). The beats are more evident at night when the patient is in a left lateral position, during or immediately following exercise and while sitting quietly (Camm & Katritsis 1996). On rare occasions the patient may experience chest pain. Sometimes the patient is asymptomatic.

Treatment

Treatment is rarely necessary (Bennett 1994). Any electrolyte imbalances should be corrected.

Interpretation of Fig. 6.1

- *QRS rate*: 70/min.
- *QRS rhythm*: slightly irregular owing to presence of junctional premature beats.
- *QRS complexes*: the junctional premature beats are of normal width and the same morphology as the

sinus beats; they occur prematurely before the next anticipated sinus beat and are followed by a compensatory pause.

- *P waves*: none associated with the junctional premature beats.
- *Relationship between P waves and QRS complexes:* no P waves associated with junctional premature beats.

The ECG in Fig. 6.1 displays sinus rhythm with junctional premature beats. The monitoring lead is lead II and the ST elevation is suggestive of acute myocardial infarction (12 lead ECG was required to help confirm this diagnosis). The absence of P waves, but normal width QRS complexes identical to those associated with the sinus beats, confirms that the ectopic focus is sited in the AV junction. The patient's blood pressure remained stable and there were no adverse affects. No treatment was required.

JUNCTIONAL ESCAPE BEATS

If the SA node fails to discharge, escape beats will normally arise from a subsidiary pacemaker, usually the AV junction. Junctional escape beats are not a primary diagnosis; they are symptomatic of an underlying primary disturbance to which they are secondary (Marriott 1988).

Following a long pause in the cardiac cycle, junctional escape beats 'rescue' the heart from cardiac standstill. To quote Marriott (1988), an escape beat 'is a rescuing beat – a friend in need – and as such, of course, should never be treated'.

The SA node usually recovers and resumes its role as pacemaker immediately following a junctional escape beat. Sometimes a series of junctional escape beats occur; six or more are commonly termed junctional escape rhythm or idiojunctional rhythm.

Junctional escape beats are characterised by late QRS complexes, which are similar in appearance to those occurring in sinus rhythm. They occur later than the expected sinus beat. They are not usually associated with retrograde conduction (Marriott 1988). It is important to distinguish between premature beats and escape beats because the latter suggests impaired pacemaker function (Bennett 1994).

Identifying features on the ECG

- *QRS rate*: determined by underlying rhythm.
- *QRS rhythm*: irregular owing to pauses.
- *QRS complexes*: usually normal width and same morphology as the QRS complexes associated with sinus beats; junctional escape beats occur later than the next anticipated sinus beat.
- *P waves*: usually absent; if present are of different morphology from those associated with sinus beats, are of opposite polarity to the QRS complexes (upright in V1 or inverted in lead II) and occur immediately prior to or following the QRS complex.
- *Relationship between P waves and QRS complexes*: if P waves present they occur immediately prior to or following the QRS complexes; if measurable, PR interval is short.

Effects on the patient

Depending on the length of the preceding pause, the patient may complain of lightheadedness or dizziness.

Treatment

Junctional escape beats themselves do not require treatment. They should not be suppressed by drugs (Bennett 1994). However, atropine is sometimes administered to speed up the underlying rhythm. Investigations may be required to establish the cause of SA node failure. Medications such as beta-blockers may need to be withdrawn or have their dose reduced. Any electrolyte imbalances should be corrected.

Interpretation of Fig. 6.2

- *QRS rate*: 50/min.
- *QRS rhythm*: irregular owing to pauses.
- *QRS complexes*: the QRS complexes in the underlying rate are wide (0.12 s/3 small squares); the junctional escape beat is of normal width and expected morphology for lead II.

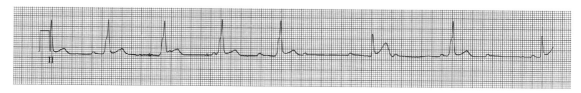

Fig. 6.2 Junctional escape beats

- *P waves*: none associated with junctional escape beat; otherwise present and constant morphology.
- *Relationship between P waves and QRS complex*: AV dissociation.

The ECG in Fig. 6.2 displays 3rd degree AV block with a ventricular escape rhythm. The ventricular rhythm is unusually rapid (50/min). However, an almost 2 s pause results in a junctional escape beat. As a rule, the inherent junctional rhythm is faster than its ventricular counterpart. On this occasion, however, it is slower, perhaps because the patient had an acute inferior myocardial infarction (increased vagal tone affecting the AV junction). No treatment was required as sinus rhythm quickly ensued.

JUNCTIONAL ESCAPE RHYTHM

Junctional escape rhythm is said to be present when there are 6 or more consecutive junctional escape beats. It can occur if the SA node fails to initiate impulses. It is not a primary diagnosis, rather a symptom of an underlying primary disturbance to which it is secondary. It is often initiated with a junctional escape beat. The inherent rate of the AV junction is 40–60 beats/min. Junctional escape rhythm begins later than the next anticipated sinus beat and the rate will be faster than the sinus rate.

Identifying features on the ECG

- *QRS rate*: usually 40–60/min.
- *QRS rhythm*: usually regular.
- *QRS complexes*: usually normal width and same configuration as the QRS complexes associated with sinus beats.
- *P waves*: usually absent; if present, are of different morphology from those associated with sinus beats, are of opposite polarity to the QRS complexes (upright in V1 or inverted in lead II) and occur immediately prior to or following the QRS complex.
- *Relationship between P waves and QRS complexes*: if P waves present they occur immediately prior to or following the QRS complexes; if measurable, PR interval is short.

Effects on the patient

The patient may be haemodynamically compromised, particularly if the rhythm is sustained. The loss of 'atrial kick' will contribute to the fall in cardiac output.

Treatment

Junctional escape rhythm itself does not require treatment. It should not be suppressed by drugs (Bennett 1994). Treatment is aimed at stimulating a higher pacemaker. Sometimes atropine is administered to speed up the underlying rhythm. Pacing may be required. The cause of SA node failure should be sought, e.g. medications, myocardial ischaemia/infarction. Any electrolyte imbalances should be corrected.

Interpretation of Fig. 6.3

- *QRS rate*: 35/min.
- *QRS rhythm*: regular.
- *QRS complexes*: normal width and morphology constant.
- *P waves*: on this lead unable to identify any P waves; a 12 lead ECG would probably highlight them situated on the T waves.
- *Relationship between P waves and QRS complexes*: not applicable.

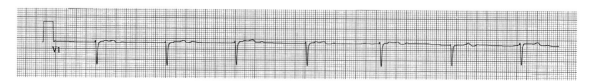

Fig. 6.3 Junctional escape rhythm

The ECG in Fig. 6.3 displays junctional escape rhythm. This patient was taking beta-blockers which may explain why the junctional rhythm is unusually slow. Although the QRS rate was slow, there were no other adverse signs. The BP was 110/70. The beta-blocker was temporarily omitted and sinus rhythm rapidly ensued. No further treatment was required.

Interpretation of Fig. 6.4

- *QRS rate*: 50/min.
- *QRS rhythm*: regular.
- *QRS complexes*: normal width and morphology constant.

- *P waves*: present but inverted.
- *Relationship between P waves and QRS complexes*: each P wave is followed by a QRS complex and each QRS complex is preceded by a P wave; abnormally short PR interval together with inverted (instead of expected upright) P waves implying retrograde conduction of the atria from the AV junction.

The ECG in Fig. 6.4 (lead II) displays junctional escape rhythm. Inverted P waves in lead II, together with a short PR interval, are characteristic ECG features of junctional escape rhythm. This patient had been admitted with a suspected myocardial infarction.

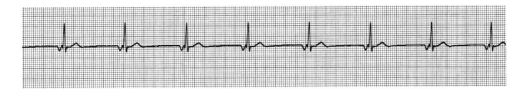

Fig. 6.4 Junctional escape rhythm

There were no adverse signs and the BP was 115/80. No treatment was required. Continuous cardiac monitoring was started.

JUNCTIONAL TACHYCARDIA

Junctional tachycardia is characterised by a sudden onset, an abrupt end, a regular rhythm and a rate of 180–200 beats/min (Camm & Katritsis 1996). The QRS complexes are of the same morphology as those associated with sinus beats (unless there is aberrant conduction or an existing conduction defect).

Tachycardia-related ST depression is frequently evident, which may persist following the termination of the arrhythmia, but is not significant (Nolan *et al.* 1998). Abnormal (retrograde) P waves may be present. However, in the majority of cases, atrial and ventricular depolarisation occurs simultaneously, with the resultant P waves either superimposed on, or hidden in, the QRS complexes.

Junctional tachycardia is normally caused by a re-entry mechanism, triggered activity or enhanced automaticity (Camm & Katritsis 1996).

Identifying features on the ECG

- *QRS rate*: usually 180–200/min.
- *QRS rhythm*: usually regular.
- *QRS complexes*: usually normal width and same morphology as the QRS complexes associated with sinus beats (unless aberrant conduction present).
- *P waves*: usually absent; if present they will be of different morphology from those associated with sinus beats and will usually be of opposite polarity to the QRS complexes (upright in V1 or inverted in lead II) and will be located immediately prior to or following the QRS complex.
- *Relationship between P waves and QRS complexes*: if P waves present they occur immediately prior to or following the QRS complexes; if measurable, PR interval is short.

Effects on the patient

Some patients may be asymptomatic. Most will complain of palpitations. Occasionally the patient may become haemodynamically compromised. This is influenced by the rate, duration of the episode and underlying cardiac disease (Wang *et al*. 1991).

Treatment

Vagal manoeuvres may slow or terminate junctional tachycardia. Adenosine is often the first drug of choice if there are no contraindications. Atrial pacing and cardioversion are other options if drug therapy fails (Nolan *et al*. 1998). If the patient is severely compromised and there are adverse signs or if other treatments fail, synchronised cardioversion is usually undertaken. Radio frequency ablation may sometimes be required (Nolan *et al*. 1998). Any electrolyte imbalances should be corrected.

Interpretation of Fig. 6.5

- *QRS rate*: 150/min.
- *QRS rhythm*: regular.
- *QRS complexes*: normal width and morphology constant.
- *P waves*: appear to be superimposed on the T waves

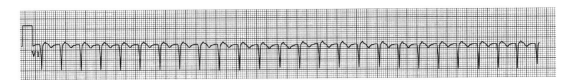

Fig. 6.5 Junctional tachycardia

immediately following the QRS complexes, opposite polarity to the QRS complexes; P waves upright in V1.
- *Relationship between P waves and QRS complexes*: P waves appear to follow QRS complexes (retrograde conduction); PR interval non-existent.

The ECG in Fig. 6.5 displays junctional tachycardia. Upright P waves in V1 (retrograde conduction from the AV junction) which are of opposite polarity to the QRS complexes (antegrade conduction from the AV junction) help to confirm the diagnosis. This patient was complaining of palpitations but was not haemodynamically compromised. The BP was 135/90 and there were no adverse signs present. The tachycardia did not respond to carotid sinus massage. However, following administration of adenosine, it did revert to sinus rhythm.

WOLFF–PARKINSON–WHITE SYNDROME

Pre-excitation can be defined as activation of the ventricle by an atrial impulse earlier than would be expected if conduction occurred via the normal AV conduction pathway (Camm & Katritsis 1996). The term was first used to describe the Wolff–Parkinson–White (WPW) syndrome. Ventricular pre-excitation produces the typical delta wave, which can be identified in sinus rhythm.

WPW syndrome is the commonest cause of an AV re-entrant tachycardia (Esberger *et al.* 2002). Thought to be hereditary (Vidaillet *et al.* 1987), its incidence is 0.1–3.7 per 1000 population (Josephson 1993).

An accessory pathway (bundle of Kent), in addition to the AV node and junction, connects the atria to the ventricles. Sometimes more than one accessory pathway is present (Colavita *et al.* 1987). The presence of an accessory pathway(s) allows the formation of a re-entry circuit, which can give rise to either a narrow complex or a broad complex tachycardia depending on whether the AV node or the accessory pathway is used for antegrade conduction (Esberger *et al.* 2002).

Identifying ECG features

Characteristic ECG features include short PR interval (< 0.12s or 3 small squares), wide QRS complex (> 0.12s or 3 small squares) with an initial delta wave and paroxysmal tachycardia (Wolff *et al.* 1930).

In sinus rhythm the atrial impulse is conducted rapidly down to the ventricles via the accessory pathway (it is not subjected to the normal delay as would be encountered in the AV node): hence the short PR interval. However, once the impulse reaches the ventricular myocardium, initially it is conducted (slowly) through non-specialised conduction tissue, distorting the early part of the R wave producing the characteristic delta wave (Esberger *et al.* 2002).

WPW syndrome has traditionally been classified into two types (A and B) according to the ECG morphology of in leads V1 and V2 (Rosenbaum *et al.* 1945):

- *Type A*: left-sided pathway resulting in a predominant R wave (Fig. 6.6)
- *Type B*: right-sided pathway resulting in a predominant S or QS wave (Fig. 6.7)

Algorithms for the localisation of overt accessory pathways, which examine the polarity of the QRS

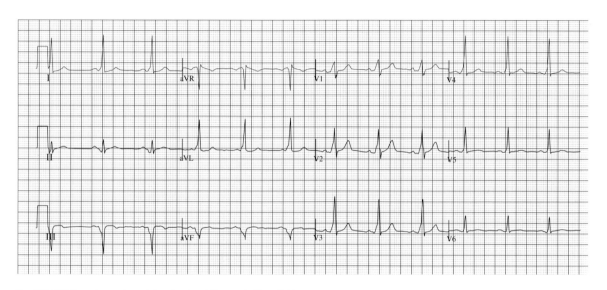

Fig. 6.6 WPW syndrome, type A (predominant R wave in V_1 and V_2)

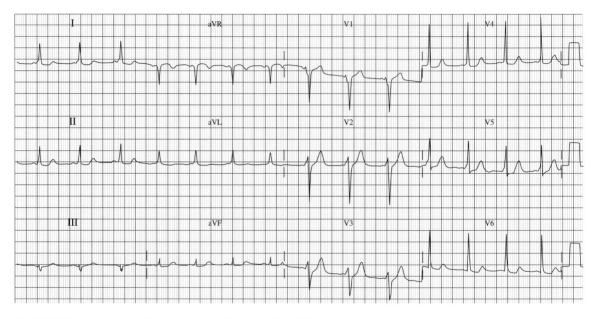

Fig. 6.7 WPW syndrome, type B (predominant S or QS wave in V_1 and V_2)

complexes, have also been proposed (Camm & Katritsis 1996).

If the accessory pathway is capable only of retrograde conduction, pre-excitation will not occur during sinus rhythm and the ECG will be normal (Esberger *et al.* 2002).

The frequency of paroxysmal tachycardia associated with WPW syndrome increases with age (Zipes 1992). If atrial fibrillation is present the ventricular response depends on the antegrade refractory period of the accessory pathway and may exceed 300/min resulting in ventricular fibrillation (Sharma *et al.* 1987).

Treatment

Patients who are symptomatic (palpitations or syncope) should be referred for electrophysiology studies (Davis 1997). Catheter ablation, which is usually done at the same time, is highly effective in the treatment of WPW syndrome (Langberg *et al.* 1992).

Drugs that block the AV node, e.g. digoxin, verapamil and adenosine, are particularly dangerous in WPW syndrome in the presence of atrial fibrillation. They decrease the refractoriness of the accessory pathways and increase the frequency of conduction, resulting in a rapid ventricular response which may lead to ventricular fibrillation (Esberger *et al.* 2002).

CHAPTER SUMMARY

Junctional arrhythmias, which originate in the AV junction, are caused by increased automaticity, suppression of the SA node, re-entry mechanisms or blocking of the impulses in the AV junction itself. Characteristics of junctional arrhythmias include narrow QRS complexes and P waves that are either absent or, if present immediately precede or follow the QRS complexes, are usually inverted in leads where they are normally upright and are of opposite polarity to the associated QRS complexes.

REFERENCES

Bennett, D.H. (1994) *Cardiac Arrhythmias*, 4th edn. Butterworth Heinemann, Oxford.

Camm, A. & Katritsis, D. (1996) The diagnosis of tachy-arrhythmias, in Julian, D. *et al.* (eds) *Diseases of the Heart*, 2nd edn. W.B. Saunders, London.

Colavita, P., Packer, D., Pressley, J. *et al.* (1987) Frequency, diagnosis and clinical characteristics of patients with multiple accessory pathways. *American Journal of Cardiology* **59**: 601.

Davis, M. (1997) Catheter ablation therapy of arrhythmias, in Thompson, P. (ed.) *Coronary Care Manual*. Churchill Livingstone, London.

Esberger, D., Jones, S. & Morris, F. (2002) ABC of clinical electrocardiography: junctional tachycardias. *British Medical Journal* **324**: 662–5.

Guyton, A. (1992) *Human Physiology and Mechanisms of Disease*, 5th edn. W.B. Saunders, Philadelphia.

Josephson, M. (1993) Pre-excitation syndromes, in Mark, E., Josephson, M.D. *Clinical Cardiac Electrophysiology*. Williams & Wilkins, London.

Langberg, J., Kalkins, H., Kim, Y. *et al.* (1992) Recurrence of conduction in accessory atrioventricular connections after initially successful radiofrequency catheter ablation. *J Am Coll Cardiol*; **19**: 1588–92.

Marriott, H.J.L. (1988) *Practical Electrocardiography*, 8th edn. Williams & Wilkins, London.

Nolan, J., Greenwood, J. & Mackintosh, A. (1998) *Cardiac Emergencies: A Pocket Guide*. Butterworth Heinemann, Oxford.

Rosenbaum, F., Hecht, H., Wilson, F. *et al.* (1945) The potential variations of the thorax and the esophagus in anomalous atrioventricular conduction (Wolff–Parkinson–White syndromes). *American Heart Journal* **29**: 281.

Sharma, A., Yee, R., Guiraudon, G. & Klein, G. (1987) Sensitivity and specificity of invasive and non-invasive testing for risk of sudden death in Wolff–Parkinson–White syndrome. *J Am Coll Cardiol*; **10**: 373.

Thompson, P. (1997) *Coronary Care Manual*. Churchill Livingstone, London.

Vidaillett, J., Pressley, J., Henke, E. *et al.* (1987) Familial occurrence of accessory atrioventricular pathways (pre-excitation syndrome). *New Englend Journal Medicine* **317**: 65.

Wang, Y., Scheinman, M., Chien, W. *et al.* (1991) Patients with supraventricular tachycardia presenting with aborted sudden death: incidence, mechanism and long-term follow-up. *J Am Coll Cardiol*; **18**: 1711.

Wolff, L., Parkinson, J., & White, D. (1930) Bundle branch block with short PR interval in healthy young people prone to paroxysmal tachycardia. *American Heart Journal* **5**: 685.

Zipes, D. (1992) Specific arrhythmias: diagnosis and treatment, in Braunwald, E. (ed.) *Heart Disease*. W.B. Saunders, Philadelphia.

Cardiac Arrhythmias Originating in the Ventricles

7

INTRODUCTION

Cardiac arrhythmias originating in the ventricles are commonly caused by an acute myocardial infarction or myocardial ischaemia. Many patients with ischaemic heart disease first present with a ventricular tachyarrhythmia, leading to cardiac arrest and sudden death, without any obvious preceding history of myocardial infarction or angina (Nolan *et al.* 1998). Other causes of ventricular arrhythmias include cardiac surgery, valvular disease, left ventricular failure, cardiomyopathy and ventricular aneurysm (Bigger 1991).

The altered pathway of impulse conduction and ventricular depolarisation associated with ventricular arrhythmias results in characteristically wide and bizarre QRS complexes which differ in morphology to QRS complexes associated with the underlying rhythm.

The aim of this chapter is to recognise cardiac arrhythmias originating in the ventricles. Ventricular fibrillation, a cardiac arrhythmia associated with cardiac arrest, is discussed in Chapter 9.

LEARNING OBJECTIVES

At the end of the chapter the reader will be able to discuss the characteristic ECG features, list the causes and outline the treatment of:

❏ ventricular premature beats;
❏ ventricular escape beats;

❏ idioventricular rhythm;
❏ accelerated idioventricular rhythm;
❏ ventricular tachycardia;
❏ 'torsades de points'.

VENTRICULAR PREMATURE BEATS

Ventricular premature beats (VPBs) are caused by an ectopic focus in the ventricles. Causes of VPBs include ischaemic heart disease, myocardial infarction, electrolyte imbalances and heart failure.

Most VPBs are wide (0.12 s/3 small squares or more) and bizarre in shape. VPB morphology differs from that of the QRS complexes associated with the underlying rhythm. Generally, a VPB originating in the left ventricle has a right bundle branch block appearance (positive in V1), and one originating in the right ventricle has a left bundle branch block appearance (negative in V1). The ST segment usually slopes in a direction opposite to the QRS deflection (Camm & Katritsis 1996). A conducted retrograde P wave may be identifiable in the ST segment/T wave. A full com-pensatory pause will usually follow a VPB – the term 'compensatory pause' is so called because the cycle following the VPB compensates for its prematurity and the sinus rhythm then resumes on schedule (Marriott 1988).

- *Uniform or unifocal VPBs*: VPBs of the same morphology (Fig. 7.1).
- *Multiform*: two or more VPBs of distinctly different morphology (the use of the term 'multifocal' is not recommended because impulses from the same focus may be conducted differently (Camm & Katritsis 1996) (Fig. 7.2).
- *R on T VPB*: a VPB which 'lands' on the T wave.
- *Ventricular bigeminy*: a VPB after every sinus beat.
- *Ventricular trigeminy*: a VPB after every two sinus beats.
- *Couplets*: pairs of VPBs (Fig. 7.3).
- *Salvos*: three or more consecutive VPBs.

Identifying features on the ECG

- *QRS rate*: determined by the underlying rhythm.
- *QRS rhythm*: irregular due to presence of VPBs.
- *QRS complexes*: wide (0.12 s/3 small squares or more), bizarre with changing amplitude, morphology and deflection; VPB morphology differs from that of the QRS complexes associated with the underlying rhythm; ST segment usually slopes in a direction opposite to the QRS deflection; occur before the next anticipated sinus beat and are usually followed by a compensatory pause.
- *P waves*: usually none associated with VPBs (situated on the T wave if present – retrograde conduction).
- *Relationship between P waves and QRS complexes*: usually not possible to determine.

Effects on the patient

The patient is usually aware of the premature beat itself, of the subsequent pause often described as a missed beat, or of a stronger post-ectopic beat (Camm & Katritsis 1996). VPBs are more evident at night when the patient is in a left lateral position, during or immediately following exercise and while sitting quietly (Camm & Katritsis 1996). On rare occasions the patient may experience chest pain. Sometimes the patient is asymptomatic.

VPBs can be associated with a significant fall in stroke volume and are often not pulse-producing. Frequent VPBs can therefore have significant haemodynamic effects on the patient.

Treatment

In the 1980s the administration of anti-arrhythmic drugs to suppress VPBs and 'prevent ventricular fibrillation' was common practice. However, the prophylactic treatment of VPBs was found to be ineffective and may in fact worsen mortality (MacMahon *et al.* 1988). It is now standard practice to treat ventricular fibrillation if it occurs rather than attempt to suppress the VPBs and prevent it. Treatable causes such as electrolyte imbalances and hypoxia should be corrected (Jowett & Thompson 1995).

Current recommendations for the management of frequent VPBs associated with acute myocardial infarction include adequate pain relief, effective treatment of heart failure and correction of any electrolyte imbalance (Nolan *et al.* 1998).

Interpretation of Fig. 7.1

- *QRS rate*: underlying rate is 60/min.
- *QRS rhythm*: irregular owing to presence of VPBs.
- *QRS complexes*: VPBs are wide (0.14 s/3.5 small squares) and bizarre; VPB morphology differs from that of the QRS complexes associated with the underlying rhythm and ST segment slopes in an opposite direction to the QRS deflection; VPBs occur before the next anticipated sinus beat and are followed by a full compensatory pause.
- *P waves*: none associated with VPBs.
- *Relationship between P waves and QRS complexes*: unable to determine.

The ECG in Fig. 7.1 displays sinus rhythm with uniform or unifocal VPBs. The VPBs have identical morphology indicating that they have been caused by

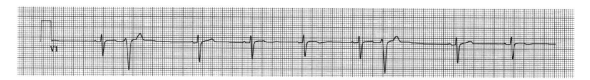

Fig. 7.1 Ventricular premature beats

the same ectopic focus in the ventricles. The patient had complained of palpitations. Only isolated VPBs were identified on the ECG and no treatment was required. The BP remained stable and there were no adverse signs. The electrolyte levels were within normal limits.

Interpretation of Fig. 7.2

- *QRS rate*: underlying rate is 80/min.
- *QRS rhythm*: slightly irregular owing to presence of VPBs.
- *QRS complexes*: VPBs are wide (0.14 s/3.5 small squares) and bizarre; VPB morphology differs from that of the QRS complexes associated with the underlying rhythm and ST segment slopes in an opposite direction to the QRS deflection; VPBs occur before the next anticipated sinus beat and are followed by a full compensatory pause.
- *P waves*: none associated with VPBs.
- *Relationship between P waves and QRS complexes*: unable to determine.

The ECG in Fig. 7.2 displays sinus rhythm with multiform VPBs. The two VPBs have varying morphology suggesting that they have been caused by two

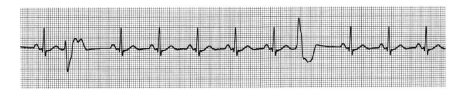

Fig. 7.2 Ventricular premature beats

ectopic foci in the ventricles. The patient's serum potassium was found to be 2.9 mmol. Following a potassium infusion the VPBs stopped occurring.

Interpretation of Fig. 7.3

- *QRS rate*: underlying rate is approximately 50/min.
- *QRS rhythm*: irregular due to presence of VPBs.
- *QRS complexes*: VPBs are wide (0.14 s/3.5 small squares) and bizarre; VPB morphology differs from that of the QRS complexes associated with the underlying rhythm and ST segment slopes in an opposite direction to the QRS deflection; VPBs occur before the next anticipated sinus beat and are followed by a full compensatory pause; some VPBs occur in pairs (couplets).
- *P waves*: none associated with VPBs.
- *Relationship between P waves and QRS complexes*: unable to determine.

The ECG in Fig. 7.3 displays sinus bradycardia with unifocal VPBs and couplets of VPBs. The VPBs have identical morphology indicating that they have been caused by the same ectopic focus in the ventricles. The patient had been admitted to CCU with a history of

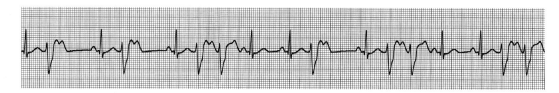

Fig. 7.3 Couplets of ventricular premature beats

chest pain. Adverse signs were present: the BP had fallen to 80/60 and he was feeling light-headed. Oxygen was administered and the patient placed in a semi-recumbent position. Atropine 500 mcg was administered i.v. in an attempt to speed up the sinus rate, which would then hopefully result in a diminished frequency of VPBs. Sinus rhythm quickly ensued and the VPBs stopped. The patient's serum electrolytes were within normal ranges. No further treatment was required.

VENTRICULAR ESCAPE BEATS

Ventricular escape beats occur if all potential pacemakers above the ventricles fail to initiate impulses or if these impulses are blocked and fail to reach the ventricles.

Ventricular escape beats are not a primary diagnosis; they are symptomatic of some underlying primary disturbance to which they are secondary (Marriott 1988). Ventricular escape beats can occur in a variety of settings, including myocardial infarction, digoxin toxicity, overdose of calcium channel blockers or beta-blockers and electrolyte disturbances (Purcell 1993).

In contrast to VPBs, ventricular escape beats occur later than the next anticipated PQRS complex associated with the underlying rhythm. Following a long pause in the underlying rhythm, ventricular escape beats 'rescue' the heart from cardiac standstill. To quote Marriott (1988), an escape beat 'is a rescuing beat – a friend in need – and as such, of course, should never be treated'.

Ventricular escape beats have similar morphological characteristics to VPBs. Most are wide (0.12 s/3 small squares or more) and bizarre in shape. VPB morphology differs from that of the QRS complexes associated with the underlying rhythm. In general, those originating in the left ventricle have a right bundle branch block appearance (positive in V1), and those originating in the right ventricle have a left bundle branch block appearance (negative in V1). The ST segment usually slopes in a direction opposite to the QRS deflection. They are not usually associated with retrograde conduction (Marriott 1988).

Normally, the SA node will recover and resume its role as pacemaker immediately following an escape beat. Sometimes a series of escape beats will occur. Six or more ventricular escape beats are commonly termed idioventricular rhythm.

Identifying features on the ECG

- *QRS rate*: determined by underlying rhythm.
- *QRS rhythm*: determined by underlying rhythm; presence of ventricular escape beats will result in pauses and an irregular rhythm.
- *QRS complexes*: usually wide (0.12 s/3 small squares or more) and bizarre, VPB morphology differs from that of the QRS complexes associated with the underlying rhythm; ST segment usually slopes in an opposite direction to the QRS deflection occur later than the next anticipated beat, i.e. following a pause in the underlying rhythm.
- *P waves*: usually absent.

- *Relationship between P waves and QRS complexes*: unable to determine.

Effects on the patient

If there are long pauses the patient may become haemodynamically compromised. The patient may be aware of the pauses.

Treatment

Ventricular escape beats themselves do not require treatment. They should not be suppressed by drugs (Bennett 1994). However, atropine is sometimes administered to speed up the underlying rhythm. Pacing may be required. The cause of SA node and junctional failure should be established and if possible treated. Any electrolyte imbalance should be corrected.

IDIOVENTRICULAR RHYTHM

An idioventricular rhythm is a series of five or more consecutive ventricular escape beats. It can occur if all potential pacemakers above the ventricles fail to initiate impulses, if the underlying rhythm is slower than the intrinsic ventricular rhythm or if there is 3rd degree AV block. The latter is the most common cause (Purcell 1993).

Idioventricular rhythm is not a primary diagnosis, rather a symptom of an underlying primary disturbance to which it is secondary. Causes include acute myocardial infarction, reperfusion following thrombolysis, drugs and electrolyte disturbances. The morphology of the QRS complexes is the same as ventricular escape beats. It is often initiated with a ventricular escape beat.

Identifying features on the ECG

- *QRS rate*: usually 20–40/min.
- *QRS rhythm*: usually regular.
- *QRS complexes*: usually wide (0.12 s/3 small squares or more) and bizarre; VPB morphology differs from that of the QRS complexes associated with the underlying rhythm; ST segment usually slopes in an opposite direction to the QRS deflection; usually starts after a pause in the underlying rhythm.
- *P waves*: usually absent, though may be present if complete AV block exists.
- *Relationship between P waves and QRS complexes*: AV dissociation if AV block present.

Effects on the patient

The patient may be haemodynamically compromised, particularly if the rhythm is sustained or slow. The loss of 'atrial kick' will contribute to the fall in cardiac output; however, it is rarely sustained.

Treatment

Idioventricular rhythm itself does not require treatment. It should not be suppressed by drugs (Bennett 1994). Treatment is aimed at stimulating a higher pacemaker. Sometimes atropine is administered to speed up the underlying rhythm. Pacing may be required. The cause of SA node and junctional failure should be established and treated if possible. Any electrolyte imbalances should be corrected.

Interpretation of Fig. 7.4

- *QRS rate*: 30/min.
- *QRS rhythm*: regular.
- *QRS complexes*: wide (0.16 s/4 small squares) and bizarre; ST segment slopes in an opposite direction to the QRS deflection.
- *P waves*: absent.
- *Relationship between P waves and QRS complexes*: unable to determine.

The ECG in Fig. 7.4 displays idioventricular rhythm. The slow rate distinguishes it from accelerated idioventricular rhythm. This patient was admitted with an acute inferior myocardial infarction. His BP was 70/45 and he was pale and clammy. As adverse signs were present, atropine 500 mcg was administered i.v. which was successful in speeding up the sinus rate. Idioventricular rhythms associated with inferior myocardial infarction rarely require treatment. However, on this occasion treatment was required because the patient was severely haemodynamically compromised.

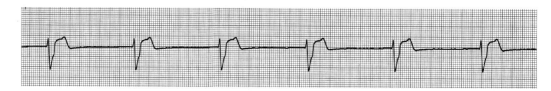

Fig. 7.4 Idioventricular rhythm

ACCELERATED IDIOVENTRICULAR RHYTHM

An accelerated idioventricular rhythm is when an ectopic ventricular focus is discharging at a rate of approximately 60–120/min. It is often caused by increased automaticity. AV dissociation is often present until the sinus rate increases sufficiently to regain control of cardiac contraction.

It is frequently associated with myocardial infarction (Lichstein *et al*. 1976; Nolan *et al*. 1998; Hampton 2000). It is also often seen during coronary reperfusion following thrombolytic therapy (Miller *et al*. 1986).

It is very similar to idioventricular rhythm except that the rate is faster and AV dissociation is often present.

Identifying features on the ECG

- *QRS rate*: 60–120/min.
- *QRS rhythm*: usually regular.
- *QRS complexes*: usually wide (0.12 s/3 small squares or more) and bizarre; VPB morphology differs from that of the QRS complexes associated with the underlying rhythm; ST segment usually slopes in an opposite direction to the QRS deflection.
- *P waves*: often present.
- *Relationship between P waves and QRS complexes*: usually AV dissociation.

Effects on the patient

An accelerated idioventricular rhythm is normally well tolerated by the patient. It is rarely associated with haemodynamic compromise and rarely degenerates into a life-threatening ventricular tachyarrhythmia (Nolan *et al*. 1998).

Treatment

An accelerated idioventricular rhythm is benign and should not be treated (Hampton 2000).

VENTRICULAR TACHYCARDIA

Ventricular tachycardia (VT) is commonly associated with ischaemic heart disease, particularly as an early or late consequence of myocardial infarction (Wellens *et al.* 1976; Josephson *et al.* 1978). During the acute phase of myocardial infarction, VT commonly deteriorates into ventricular fibrillation and is responsible for a considerable number of sudden cardiac deaths in the community (Camm & Katritsis 1996). Other causes of VT include cardiomyopathy, electrolyte imbalances and drugs.

VT is diagnosed if there are five or more QRS complexes (Camm & Katritsis 1996). It is classed as sustained VT if it lasts for more than 30 seconds and unsustained VT if it lasts for less than 30 seconds (Josephson 1993; Edhouse & Morris 2002). The QRS complexes are wide (0.12 s/3 small squares or more) and bizarre. Monomorphic VT is when the QRS complexes are of constant shape. Polymorphic VT is when the QRS morphology changes ('torsades de points', an important variety of this, is discussed in the next section).

In approximately 70% of cases of VT, the atria may continue to depolarise independently of the ventricle, i.e. AV dissociation (Camm & Katritsis 1996). As this activity is completely independent of ventricular activity, the resultant P waves are dissociated from the QRS complexes and are positive in lead II (Edhouse & Morris 2002). This independent atrial activity can lead to fusion and capture beats, the presence of which are hallmarks of ventricular tachycardia.

A fusion beat is when an impulse from the SA node travelling antegradely meets an impulse from the ventricles travelling retrogradely. The ventricles are therefore depolarised partly by the impulse being conducted through the His–Purkinje system and partly by the impulse arising in the ventricle (Edhouse & Morris 2002). The QRS complex that results partly resembles a normal complex and partly resembles a VPB complex (Jowett & Thompson 1995). Fusion beats are uncommon, and although their presence supports a diagnosis of ventricular tachycardia, their absence does not exclude the diagnosis (Edhouse & Morris 2002).

A capture beat is when an impulse from the SA node

is conducted to the ventricles resulting in a P wave followed by a normal QRS complex (Jowett & Thompson 1995), without otherwise interrupting the arrhythmia (Resuscitation Council UK 2000). Capture beats are uncommon, and although their presence supports a diagnosis of ventricular tachycardia, their absence does not exclude the diagnosis (Edhouse & Morris 2002).

Most broad complex tachycardias are ventricular in origin, i.e. ventricular tachycardia. Occasionally a supraventricular tachycardia can be conducted with bundle branch block resulting in a broad complex tachycardia. Twelve lead ECGs should be recorded whenever possible to help confirm diagnosis.

Identifying features on the ECG

- *QRS rate*: usually 150–200/min.
- *QRS rhythm*: regular or irregular.
- *QRS complexes*: wide (0.12 s/3 small squares or more) and bizarre; VPB morphology differs from the QRS complexes associated with the underlying rhythm; ST segment usually slopes in a direction opposite to the QRS deflection.
- *P waves*: may be present.
- *Relationship between P waves and QRS complexes*: if P waves visible, AV dissociation is often present.

Effects on the patient

Ventricular tachycardia is a serious cardiac arrhythmia. The patient will often be haemodynamically compromised. In some patients cardiac output will be lost. It can degenerate into ventricular fibrillation.

Treatment

If the patient is pulseless, immediate defibrillation is required. If the patient has a pulse but is haemodynamically compromised, early cardioversion is advocated. If the patient is stable pharmaceutical therapy such as amiodarone or lidocaine (lignocaine) are recommended (Resuscitation Council UK 2000). Any underlying causes, e.g. electrolyte imbalances, should be treated if possible.

Interpretation of Fig. 7.5

- *QRS rate*: 150/min.
- *QRS rhythm*: regular.
- *QRS complexes*: wide (0.14 s/3.5 small squares) and bizarre, ST segment slopes in a direction opposite to the QRS deflection.
- *P waves*: some identifiable.
- *Relationship between P waves and QRS complexes*: AV dissociation is present – there is no relationship between the P waves and QRS complexes.

The ECG in Fig. 7.5 displays a broad complex tachycardia which is most likely to be ventricular in origin, i.e. ventricular tachycardia. This patient was stable. His BP was 120/70 and he was well perfused. The ventricular rate is only a borderline adverse sign (Resuscitation Council UK 2000). Amiodarone infusion provided effective treatment. Fig. 11.24 on page 182 depicts a 12 lead ECG recorded in this patient.

Interpretation of Fig. 7.6

- *QRS rate*: 200/min.
- *QRS rhythm*: regular.
- *QRS complexes*: wide (0.12 s/3 small squares) and bizarre; ST segment slopes in a direction opposite to the QRS deflection.
- *P waves*: not identifiable.

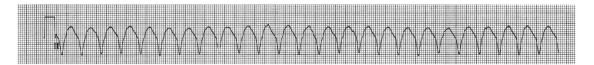

Fig. 7.5 Ventricular tachycardia

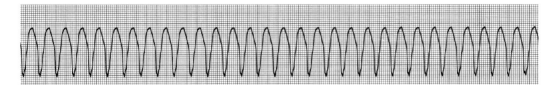

Fig. 7.6 Ventricular tachycardia

- *Relationship between P waves and QRS complexes*: unable to determine.

The ECG in Fig. 7.6 displays a broad complex tachycardia most likely ventricular in origin. A 12 lead ECG would be required to confirm diagnosis. This patient had been admitted to A&E with acute anterior myocardial infarction. He was severely compromised and adverse signs were present. His BP was unrecordable and the patient was semi-conscious. In addition, the rate is very rapid and there is a high risk of degeneration into cardiac arrest. Urgent treatment was required. Synchronised cardioversion was carried out. Success-ful conversion to sinus rhythm was achieved on the second attempt (200 J).

TORSADES DE POINTS

Torsades de points or 'twisting of the points' is a form of polymorphic VT. It refers to an ECG appearance of spiky QRS complexes rotating irregularly around the isoelectric line at a rate of 200–250 beats/min (Dessertenne 1966). The cardiac axis rotates over a sequence of 5–20 beats, changing from one direction to another and then back again (Edhouse & Morris 2002).

Torsades de points is usually associated with a prolonged QT interval. Causes include anti-arrhythmic drugs, bradycardia due to sick sinus syndrome or AV block, congenital prolongation of the QT interval (e.g. Romano Ward syndrome), hypokalaemia, hypomagnesaemia and tricyclic antidepressant drugs (Bennett 1994).

It is important to recognise torsades de points because the administration of anti-arrhythmic drugs (sometimes adminstered for monomorphic VT) may actually aggravate it. In addition, correction or removal of the cause may be very effective.

Although it is usually non-sustained and repetitive (Bennett 1994), it can itself cause a cardiac arrest or degenerate into ventricular fibrillation (Resuscitation Council UK 2000).

Identifying features on the ECG

- *QRS rate*: usually 200–250/min.
- *QRS rhythm*: irregular.
- *QRS complexes*: wide (0.12 s/3 small squares or more) and bizarre, with changing amplitude, morphology and deflection.
- *P waves*: unable to identify.
- *Relationship between P waves and QRS complexes*: AV dissociation may be present.

Effects on the patient

Torsades de points is a very serious cardiac arrhythmia. The patient will often be haemodynamically compromised. In some patients cardiac output will be lost. It can degenerate into ventricular fibrillation.

Treatment

Effective treatment, i.e. prevention of recurrent episodes, involves removal of any predisposing causes, e.g. drugs, correction of any electrolyte imbalances and possibly overdrive pacing (Resuscitation Council UK 2000). Measures to speed up the sinus rate may be effective in some situations. If the patient has a cardiac arrest, early defibrillation will be required.

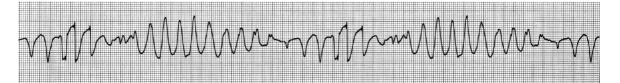

Fig. 7.7 Torsades de points

Interpretation of Fig. 7.7

- *QRS rate*: 200–250/min.
- *QRS rhythm*: irregular.
- *QRS complexes*: wide and bizarre, with changing amplitude, morphology and deflection.
- *P waves*: unable to identify.
- *Relationship between P waves and QRS complexes*: unable to determine.

CHAPTER SUMMARY

Cardiac arrhythmias originating in the ventricles are characterised by wide, bizarre QRS complexes. Most ventricular tachyarrhythmias are serious. Some can have severe haemodynamic effects on the patient whereas others can cause a cardiac arrest. Their prompt recognition together with appropriate treatment is essential.

REFERENCES

Bennett, D.H. (1994) *Cardiac Arrhythmias*, 4th edn. Butterworth Heinemann, Oxford.

Bigger, J. (1991) Ventricular dysrhythmias, in Horowitz, L. (ed.) *Current Management of Arrhythmias*. B.C. Decker, Philadelphia.

Camm, A. & Katritsis, D. (1996) The diagnosis of tachyarrhythmias, in Julian, D. *et al.* (eds) *Diseases of the Heart* 2nd edn. W.B. Saunders, London.

Dessertenne, F. (1966) La tachycardie ventriculaire a deux foyers opposes variables. *Arch Mal Coeur* **59**: 263.

Edhouse, J. & Morris, F. (2002) ABC of clinical electrocardiography: broad complex tachycardia – part 2. *British Medical Journal* **324**: 776–9.

Hampton, J. (2000) *The ECG Made Easy*, 5th edn. Churchill Livingstone, London.

Josephson, M. (1993) *Clinical Cardiac Electrophysiology*. Lea & Febiger, Philadelphia.

Josephson, M., Horowitz, L., Farsidi, A. & Kastor, J. (1978) Recurrent sustained ventricular tachycardia: 1. Mechanisms. *Circulation* **57**: 431.

Jowett, N.I. & Thompson, D.R. (1995) *Comprehensive Coronary Care*, 2nd edn. Scutari Press, London.

Lichstein, E., Ribas-Meneclier, C., Gupta, P. & Chadda, A. (1976) Incidence and descriptions of accelerated idioventricular rhythm complicating acute myocardial infarction. *American Journal of Medicine* **58**: 192–8.

MacMahon, S., Collins, R., Peto, R. *et al.* (1988) Effects of prophylactic lidocaine in suspected myocardial infarction. An overview of results from the randomized controlled trials. *JAMA* **2601**: 1910–16.

Marriott, H.J.L. (1988) *Practical Electrocardiography*, 8th edn. Williams & Wilkins, London.

Miller, F., Kruchoff, M., Satler, L. *et al.* (1986) Ventricular arrhythmias during reperfusion, *American Heart Journal* **112**: 928–31.

Nolan, J., Greenwood, J. & Mackintosh, A. (1998) *Cardiac Emergencies: A Pocket Guide*. Butterworth Heinemann, Oxford.

Purcell, J. (1993) Cardiac electrical activity, in Kinney, M., Packa, D. & Dunbar, S. (eds) *AACN's Clinical Reference for Critical Care Nursing*, 3rd edn. Mosby–Year Book, St Louis.

Resuscitation Council UK (2000) *Advanced Life Support Manual*, 4th edn. Resuscitation Council UK, London.

Wellens, H., Durer, D. & Lie, K. (1976) Observation on mechanisms of ventricular tachycardia in man. *Circulation* **54**: 327.

Cardiac Arrhythmias with Atrioventricular Block

8

INTRODUCTION

Cardiac arrhythmias with atrioventricular (AV) block can result from a conduction disturbance in the AV node, Bundle of His or bundle branches. It is classified as 1st, 2nd or 3rd degree depending on whether impulse conduction to the ventricles is delayed, intermittently blocked or completely blocked (Bennett 1994).

Normally, a narrow QRS complex indicates a conduction disturbance in the AV node or Bundle of His, whereas a wide QRS complex indicates a conduction disturbance in the bundle branches.

The aim of this chapter is to recognise cardiac arrhythmias with AV block.

LEARNING OBJECTIVES

At the end of the chapter the reader will be able to state the characteristic ECG features, list the causes and outline the treatment of:

❏ first degree AV block;
❏ second degree AV block Mobitz type 1 (Wenckeback phenomenon);
❏ second degree AV block Mobitz type 2;
❏ third degree AV block.

FIRST DEGREE AV BLOCK

First degree AV block, characterised by a prolonged PR interval (> 0.20 s or 5 small squares), signifies delayed conduction in the AV junction (AV node or Bundle of His) (Resuscitation Council UK 2000). All the impulses are conducted to the ventricles and there are no missed beats.

Although first degree AV block is not in itself important, it may be a sign of coronary heart disease, acute rheumatic carditis, digoxin toxicity or electrolyte imbalance (Hampton 2000). Sometimes it is a normal phenomenon.

Forty per cent of patients with an acute inferior myocardial infarction and 1st degree AV block, develop self-terminating well-tolerated episodes of 2nd degree AV block type 1 and 3rd degree AV block (Nolan *et al.* 1998). When associated with an anterior myocardial infarction, it may be the final stage of widespread involvement of the conduction system in septal infarction (Thompson 1997).

Identifying features on the ECG

- *QRS rate*: usually normal.
- *QRS rhythm*: usually regular.
- *QRS complexes*: normal width and morphology.
- *P waves*: present and constant morphology.
- *Relationship between P waves and QRS complexes*: each P wave is followed by a QRS complex and each QRS complex is preceded by a P wave; PR interval is prolonged, i.e. > 0.20 s/5 small squares.

Effects on the patient

The patient will be asymptomatic. First degree AV block does not alter the ventricular rate and the abnormality can only be detected on the ECG (Jowett & Thompson 1995).

Treatment

It requires no specific treatment, apart from avoiding drugs which may prolong AV conduction, e.g. beta-blockers. However, it is important to monitor the patient closely in case there is progression to a higher degree of AV block.

Interpretation of Fig. 8.1

- *QRS rate*: 80/min.
- *QRS rhythm*: regular.
- *QRS complexes*: normal width and morphology.
- *P waves*: present and constant morphology.
- *Relationship between P waves and QRS complexes*: each P wave is followed by a QRS complex and each QRS complex is preceded by a P wave; PR interval is prolonged 0.22 s (6 small squares).

The ECG in Fig. 8.1 displays 1st degree AV block. It was only identified following a routine 12 lead ECG. The patient was asymptomatic and no treatment was required.

SECOND DEGREE AV BLOCK MOBITZ TYPE 1 (WENCKEBACK PHENOMENON)

Second degree AV block Mobitz type 1 (Wenckeback's phenomenon), is the commonest (90%) form of this degree of AV block (Jowett & Thompson 1995). It can be caused by any condition that delays AV conduction, resulting in intermittent failure of transmission of the atrial impulse to the ventricles (Da Costa *et al.* 2002). Causes include inferior myocardial infarction (most common cause), electrolyte imbalance and drugs that suppress AV conduction, e.g. beta-blockers, digoxin and diltiazem.

When associated with an inferior myocardial infarction, it usually has a gradual onset, progressing from

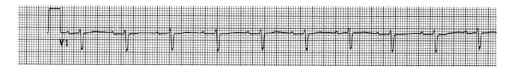

Fig. 8.1 First degree AV block

1st degree AV block over a period of hours and often leading on to 3rd degree AV block before reverting back to normal AV conduction after a further period of 2nd degree AV block (Thompson 1997). This sequence of events can be accelerated following right coronary reperfusion, as a result of the Bezold–Jarisch reflex (Koren *et al.* 1986).

It is characterised by a progressive prolongation of the PR interval until an impulse fails to be conducted to the ventricles, resulting in a dropped beat (QRS complex). This is then followed by a conducted impulse, a shorter PR interval and a repetition of the cycle (Hampton 2000). The number of dropped beats is variable. Sometimes gradual shortening of the RR interval is evident.

Identifying features on the ECG

- *QRS rate*: depending on the number of dropped beats, may be bradycardic.

- *QRS rhythm*: usually irregular (unless 2:1 conduction).
- *QRS complexes*: usually normal width and morphology.
- *P waves*: present and constant morphology, PP interval remains constant.
- *Relationship between P waves and QRS complexes*: not every P wave is followed by a QRS, but every QRS complex is preceded by a P wave; PR interval progressively lengthens until a QRS complex is dropped; RR interval progressively shortens.

Effects on the patient

The patient is rarely haemodynamically compromised, unless the ventricular rate is slow.

Treatment

Usually the only active treatment required, apart from avoiding AV junctional blocking drugs, is close monitoring of the patient (Nolan *et al.* 1998). If the ventricular rate is slow, atropine, and, rarely, cardiac pacing, may be required.

Interpretation of Fig. 8.2

- *QRS rate*: 50/min.
- *QRS rhythm*: irregular.
- *QRS complexes*: normal.
- *P waves*: present and constant morphology, PP interval remains constant.
- *Relationship between P waves and QRS complexes*: not every P wave is followed by a QRS, but every

QRS complex is preceded by a P wave; PR interval progressively lengthens until a QRS complex is dropped.

The ECG in Fig. 8.2 displays 2nd degree AV block type 1 (Wenckeback's phenomenon). It was seen in a patient with an acute inferior myocardial infarction and it followed a period of 1st degree AV block. On this occasion, because the ventricular rate was slow and the patient was haemodynamically compromised (BP 80/60 and complaining of dizziness), atropine 500 mcg i.v. was administered with effect.

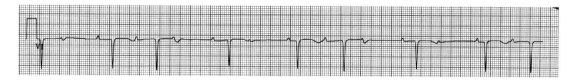

Fig. 8.2 Second degree AV block Mobitz type 1 (Wenckeback's phenomenon)

SECOND DEGREE AV BLOCK MOBITZ TYPE 2

Second degree AV block Mobitz type 2 is characterised by an intermittent failure of atrial impulse conduction to the ventricles (Bennett 1994). It is not as common as 2nd degree AV block type 1, but its implications are significantly more serious (Da Costa *et al*. 2002). The block is usually at the level of the bundle branches, commonly resulting in a wide QRS complex (Da Costa *et al*. 2002).

It is never a normal finding (Conover 1992). It is often associated with advanced cardiac disease and often progresses to 3rd degree AV block or asystole (Jowett & Thompson 1995). If 3rd degree AV block develops, it is often quite sudden and unexpected, with a slow ventricular escape rhythm and a marked deterioration in haemodynamic status (Brown *et al*. 1969). Patients with anterior myocardial infarction who develop 2nd degree AV block Mobitz type 2 have a poor prognosis (Nolan *et al*. 1998).

In 2nd degree AV block Mobitz type 2, the PR interval remains constant in the conducted beats, but some of the P waves are not followed by a QRS complex (Resuscitation Council UK 2000), i.e. there are dropped beats.

Identifying features on the ECG

- *QRS rate*: depends on the number of dropped beats; may be normal or bradycardic.
- *QRS rhythm*: usually irregular due to dropped beats (unless 2:1 conduction).
- *QRS complexes*: usually wide (0.12 s/3 small squares or more) with bundle branch block pattern, may be normal width and morphology.
- *P waves*: present and constant morphology.
- *Relationship between P waves and QRS complexes*: not every P wave is followed by a QRS complex (dropped beats); every QRS complex is preceded by a P wave; PR interval constant.

Effects on the patient

The patient is often haemodynamically compromised

(Da Costa *et al.* 2002). Progression to ventricular standstill and cardiac arrest is not uncommon.

Treatment
Prophylactic temporary pacing is usually required (Nolan *et al.* 1998).

Interpretation of Fig. 8.3

- *QRS rate*: 50–60/min.
- *QRS rhythm*: irregular due to dropped beats.
- *QRS complexes*: normal width and morphology.
- *P waves*: present and constant morphology.
- *Relationship between P waves and QRS complexes*: not every P wave is followed by a QRS complex (dropped beats); every QRS complex is preceded by a P wave, PR interval constant.

The ECG in Fig. 8.3 displays 2nd degree AV block Mobitz type 2. This patient had been admitted with an acute anterior myocardial infarction. Although the patient was haemodynamically stable, there was a risk that the arrhythmia could degenerate into 3rd degree AV block, or even ventricular standstill. Temporary cardiac pacing was required.

THIRD DEGREE AV BLOCK
Third degree AV block or complete AV block is characterised by AV dissociation – the P waves bear no

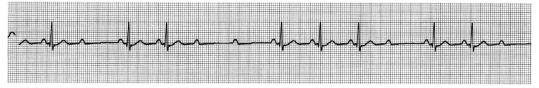

Fig. 8.3 Second degree AV block Mobitz type 2

relation to the QRS complexes and there is total independence of atrial and ventricular contractions (Da Costa *et al.* 2002). Although atrial contraction is normal, complete AV block prevents the impulses being conducted to the ventricles. The ventricular rhythm is maintained by a junctional (narrow QRS and more reliable) or ventricular escape (wide QRS and less reliable) rhythm.

It can be an acute phenomenon usually associated with a myocardial infarction or may be chronic, usually caused by fibrosis of the Bundle of His (Hampton 2000). Other causes include cardiac surgery, endocarditis and drugs (Bennett 1994). When associated with acute myocardial infarction, the pathophysiology and recommended treatment will depend on the site of the infarct (Nolan *et al.* 1998).

When associated with an inferior myocardial infarction, it is normally caused by ischaemia or necrosis of the AV node together with activation of the vagus nerve (Thompson 1997). It develops slowly, being often preceded by 1st degree and then 2nd degree AV

block Mobitz type 1 (Wenckeback). It is generally well tolerated (Nolan *et al.* 1998). The QRS complex is narrow, signifying a junctional escape rhythm which is usually reliable and of an adequate rate. Normal AV conduction usually resumes within 24 hours (Nolan *et al.* 1998).

When associated with anterior myocardial infarction, it is frequently a sudden event, especially in patients who develop 2nd degree AV block Mobitz type 2 or left bundle branch block (Nolan *et al.* 1998). There is extensive necrosis of the septum, with damage to both the left and right bundle branches (Thompson 1997). The QRS complex is wide, signifying a ventricular escape rhythm, unreliable and slow. The mortality rate in these patients is as high as 80% (Nolan *et al.* 1998).

Sometimes 3rd degree AV block is a chronic phenomenon, particularly in the elderly. The patient may be admitted following a history of falls or blackouts: a diagnosis being made following a routine 12 lead ECG.

Identifying features on the ECG

- *QRS rate*: dependent upon the site of the subsidiary pacemaker; 40–60 if junctional, < 40 if ventricular.
- *QRS rhythm*: regular.
- *QRS complexes*: may be normal (if junctional pacemaker), otherwise wide (0.12 s/3 small squares or more) with bundle branch block pattern (ventricular pacemaker).
- *P waves*: present and constant morphology, usually faster rate than the QRS complexes; absent if underlying rhythm is atrial fibrillation.
- *Relationship between P waves and QRS complexes*: AV dissociation.

Effects on the patient

Some patients will have an adequate escape rhythm that will maintain their blood pressure while others will be compromised requiring urgent intervention. Generally the effects on the patient will depend on the cause.

When associated with an anterior myocardial infarction, the patient is haemodynamically compromised. The risk of ventricular standstill and sudden cardiac arrest is high. If associated with an inferior myocardial infarction the patient may be haemodynamically stable. If chronic, the patient may present with a history of blackouts or falls.

Treatment

Again, this will depend on the cause. If associated with an inferior myocardial infarction, pacing will usually only be required if the ventricular rate is less than 40 or if the patient is haemodynamically compromised (Thompson 1997). It may respond to just atropine. If associated with an anterior myocardial infarction, a temporary and then often a permanent cardiac pacemaker will be required (ACC/AHA 1991). External pacing is a recommended interim measure (Resuscitation Council UK 2000). If chronic, a permanent pacemaker will usually be required.

Interpretation of Fig. 8.4

- *QRS rate*: 55/min.
- *QRS rhythm*: regular.
- *QRS complexes*: wide (0.12 s/3 small squares) and bizarre indicating a ventricular pacemaker.
- *P waves*: present and constant morphology, rate 60/min; some appear on the T waves and some are hidden in the QRS complexes.
- *Relationship between P waves and QRS complexes*: AV dissociation.

The ECG in Fig. 8.4 displays 3rd degree AV block. This patient had been admitted with an inferior myocardial infarction. It was preceded by 1st degree AV block and then 2nd degree AV block Mobitz type 1. It was only transient and it was well tolerated by the patient (BP 100/65). No intervention was required, except the administration of oxygen.

Interpretation of Fig. 8.5

- *QRS rate*: 30/min.
- *QRS rhythm*: regular.
- *QRS complexes*: wide (0.12 s/3 small squares) and bizarre indicating a ventricular pacemaker.
- *P waves*: present and constant morphology, rate

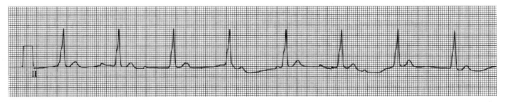

Fig. 8.4 Third degree AV block

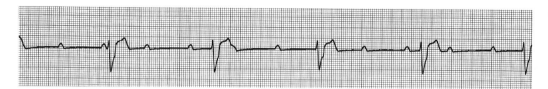

Fig. 8.5 Third degree AV block

65/min; some appear on the T waves and some are hidden in the QRS complexes.

- *Relationship between P waves and QRS complexes*: AV dissociation.

The ECG in Fig. 8.5 displays 3rd degree AV block. This patient was admitted with a history suggestive of acute myocardial infarction. His blood pressure was unrecordable. He was unconscious. The patient required urgent cardiac pacing.

CHAPTER SUMMARY

Cardiac arrhythmias with AV block can result from a conduction disturbance in the AV node, Bundle of His or bundle branches. They are classified as 1st, 2nd or 3rd degree depending on whether impulse conduction to the ventricles is delayed, intermittently blocked or completely blocked (Bennett 1994). Accurate interpretation is important because some are benign whereas others can be life-threatening.

REFERENCES

ACC/AHA (1991) Guidelines for implantation of cardiac pacemakers and anti-arrhythmic devices. A report of the ACC/AHA task force on assessment of diagnostic and therapeutic cardiovascular procedures (Committee on Pacemaker Implantation). *JACC* **18**: 1–13.

Bennett, D.H. (1994) *Cardiac Arrhythmias*, 4th edn. Butterworth Heinemann, Oxford.

Brown, R., Hunt, D. & Sloman, J. (1969) The natural history of atrioventricular conduction defects in acute myocardial infarction. *American Heart Journal* **78**: 460–6.

Conover, M. (1992) *Understanding Electrocardiography: Arrhythmias and the 12 Lead ECG*, 6th edn. Mosby–Year Book, St Louis.

Da Costa, D., Brady, W. & Redhouse, J. (2002) ABC of clinical electrocardiography: bradycardias and atrioventricular block. *British Medical Journal* **324**: 535–8.

Hampton, J. (2000) *The ECG Made Easy*, 5th edn. Churchill Livingstone, Edinburgh.

Jowett, N.I. & Thompson, D.R. (1995) *Comprehensive Coronary Care* 2nd edn. Scutari Press, London.

Koren, G., Weiss, A., Ben-David, T. *et al.* (1986) Bradycardia and hypotension following reperfusion with streptokinase (Bezold-Jarisch reflex): a sign of coronary thrombolysis and myocardial salvage. *American Heart Journal* **112**: 468–71.

Nolan, J., Greenwood, J. & Mackintosh, A. (1998) *Cardiac Emergencies: A Pocket Guide*. Butterworth Heinemann, Oxford.

Resuscitation Council UK (2000) *Advanced Life Support Manual*, 4th edn. Resuscitation Council UK, London.

Thompson, P. (1997) *Coronary Care Manual*. Churchill Livingstone, London.

Cardiac Arrhythmias Associated with Cardiac Arrest

9

INTRODUCTION

Cardiac arrhythmias associated with cardiac arrest include ventricular fibrillation (VF), pulseless ventricular tachycardia (VT), asystole, ventricular standstill, pulseless electrical activity (formally called electromechanical dissociation or EMD) and agonal rhythm. Ventricular tachycardia has been discussed in detail in Chapter 7 and will not be discussed again here.

The aim of this chapter is to recognise cardiac arrhythmias associated with cardiac arrest.

LEARNING OBJECTIVES

At the end of the chapter the reader will be able to state the characteristic ECG features of and outline the treatment for:

❑ ventricular fibrillation;

❑ asystole;

❑ ventricular standstill;

❑ pulseless electrical activity;

❑ agonal rhythm.

VENTRICULAR FIBRILLATION

'The cardiac pump is thrown out of gear, and the last of its vital energy is dissipated in a violent and prolonged turmoil of fruitless activity in the ventricular walls.'

(McWilliam 1889)

VF is the commonest primary arrhythmia at the onset of a cardiac arrest in adults (Sedgwick *et al.* 1994). It is the presenting arrhythmia in 30% of in-hospital

(Gwinnutt *et al.* 2000) and 80% of out-of-hospital cardiac arrests (Colquhoun & Jevon 2000).

An eminently treatable arrhythmia, the only effective treatment is early defibrillation and the likelihood of success is crucially time dependent (Colquhoun & Jevon 2000). Causes include ishaemic heart disease, heart failure, electrolyte imbalance, drugs, hypothermia and cardiomyopathy.

Characteristic ECG features include a bizarre irregular waveform, apparently random in both amplitude and frequency, reflecting disorganised electrical activity in the myocardium. Initially the amplitude of the waveform is coarse. However, it will rapidly deteriorate into fine VF and then asystole, reflecting the depletion of myocardial high-energy phosphate stores (Mapin *et al.* 1991).

Identifying features on the ECG

- *QRS rate*: unable to determine.
- *QRS rhythm*: unable to determine.
- *QRS complexes*: none recognisable.
- *P waves*: none recognisable.
- *Relationship between P waves and QRS complexes*: no recognisable P waves or QRS complexes present.

If there is electrical activity, but there are no recognisable complexes, the most likely diagnosis is ventricular fibrillation (Resuscitation Council UK 2000).

Effects on the patient

The patient will have a cardiac arrest.

Treatment

Confirm cardiac arrest and defibrillate immediately. If unable to defibrillate or if the defibrillator is not immediately available, start cardiopulmonary resuscitation (CPR). Consider a precordial thump in a witnessed, particularly monitored, cardiac arrest (Colquhoun & Chamberlain 1999). If delivered within 30 seconds, it may terminate VF in 2% of cases (Kerber & Robertson 1996).

Early defibrillation is the definitive treatment; the chances of success decline substantially (7–10%) for every minute it is delayed (Cobbe *et al.* 1991). Adequate CPR can slow this decline (Larsen *et al.* 1993). Forty-three per cent of patients who initially present with VF at the onset of a cardiac arrest survive to discharge (Gwinnutt *et al.* 2000).

The European Resuscitation Council guidelines for the management of ventricular fibrillation (Latorre *et al.* 2001) are depicted in Fig. 9.1.

Interpretation of Fig. 9.2

- *QRS rate*: unable to determine.
- *QRS rhythm*: unable to determine.
- *QRS complexes*: none recognisable.
- *P waves*: none recognisable.
- *Relationship between P waves and QRS complexes*: no recognisable P waves or QRS complexes present.

The ECG in Fig. 9.2 displays coarse VF. This patient was admitted to A&E with chest pain. Once cardiac arrest was confirmed, defibrillation with 200 J was carried out immediately, with success.

Interpretation of Fig. 9.3

- *QRS rate*: unable to determine.
- *QRS rhythm*: unable to determine.
- *QRS complexes*: none recognisable.
- *P waves*: none recognisable.
- *Relationship between P waves and QRS complexes*: no recognisable P waves or QRS complexes present.

The ECG in Fig. 9.3 displays fine VF. Once cardiac arrest had been confirmed, defibrillation with 200 J was undertaken twice. Asystole ensued. Fortunately, after a minute of CPR, sinus rhythm returned, together with cardiac output.

ASYSTOLE

Asystole is the presenting rhythm in approximately 25% of in-hospital cardiac arrests (Gwinnutt *et al.* 2000). In asystole, ventricular standstill is present owing to the suppression of all natural cardiac pacemakers.

Failure of sinus rhythm, under normal circumstances, will lead to the appearance of an escape

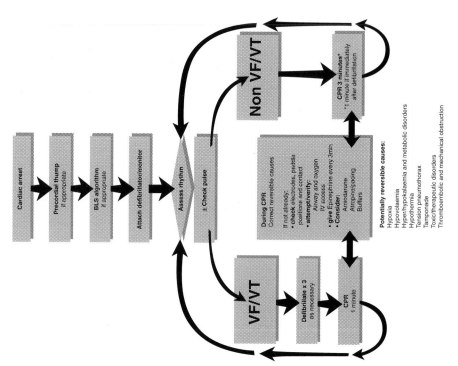

Fig. 9.1 European Resuscitation Council guidelines for adult advanced life support (reproduced by kind permission of Aurum pharmaceuticals)

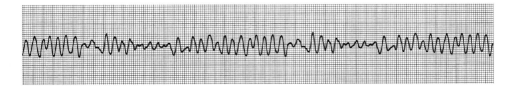

Fig. 9.2 Coarse ventricular fibrillation

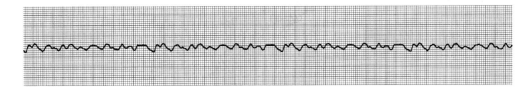

Fig. 9.3 Fine ventricular fibrillation

rhythm maintained by a subsidiary pacemaker situated in either the AV junction (junctional rhythm) or ventricular myocardium (idioventricular rhythm). Myocardial disease, hypoxia, drugs and electrolyte imbalance can all suppress these escape rhythms.

It is most important to ensure the ECG trace is accurate. Other causes of a 'flat line' ECG trace include incorrect lead and ECG gain settings, and disconnected ECG leads (Jevon 2002) (see Chapter 3). Sometimes, 'asystole' may be displayed on the monitor immediately following defibrillation, when monitoring using defibrillation paddles, regardless of the true ECG rhythm (Chamberlain 1999). This is more common following multiple shocks and where there is high chest impedance (Bradbury *et al.* 2000). If this phenomenon is encountered, the ECG leads should be used for ECG monitoring (Resuscitation Council UK 2000).

Identifying features on the ECG

- *QRS rate*: no electrical activity present.
- *QRS rhythm*: no electrical activity present.
- *QRS complexes*: no electrical activity present.
- *P waves*: no electrical activity present.
- *Relationship between P waves and QRS complexes*: no electrical activity present.

Effects on the patient

The patient will have a cardiac arrest. The prognosis is very poor. Asystole is often terminal.

Treatment

Confirm cardiac arrest, check that the rhythm is indeed asystole and not, for example, ventricular fibrillation (ECG gain, lead connections, correct lead settings on the monitor), and, if indicated, start CPR.

The European Resuscitation Council guidelines for the management of asystole (non-VF/VT) (Latorre *et al.* 2001) are depicted in Fig. 9.1 on p. 122.

Interpretation of Fig. 9.4

- *QRS rate*: no QRS complexes present.
- *QRS rhythm*: no QRS complexes present.
- *QRS complexes*: no QRS complexes present.
- *P waves*: no P waves present.
- *Relationship between P waves and QRS complexes*: no QRS complexes present.

The ECG in Fig. 9.4 displays probable asystole. Confirm cardiac arrest, check that the rhythm is indeed asystole and not, for example, ventricular fibrillation

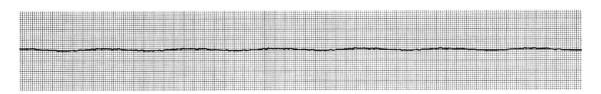

Fig. 9.4 Asystole

(ECG gain, lead connections, correct lead settings on the monitor), and, if indicated, start CPR.

VENTRICULAR STANDSTILL

Ventricular standstill is characterised by the presence of P waves and absent QRS complexes. One cause is that the sinus impulses are conducted to the ventricles, but the ventricles fail to respond to stimulation. Another cause is that they are not conducted to the ventricles because of the presence of complete AV block and an idioventricular rhythm fails to 'kick in'. Sometimes, ventricular standstill can occur quite sud-denly if the patient is already in 2nd degree AV block Mobitz type 2 or 3rd degree AV block.

Identifying features on the ECG

- *QRS rate*: no QRS complexes present.
- *QRS rhythm*: no QRS complexes present.
- *QRS complexes*: no QRS complexes present.
- *P waves*: present.
- *Relationship between P waves and QRS complexes*: no QRS complexes present.

Effects on the patient

The patient will have a cardiac arrest.

Treatment

Confirm cardiac arrest and start CPR and emergency pacing (external initially if facilities available, and then transvenous).

The European Resuscitation Council guidelines for the management of ventricular standstill (non-VF/VT) (Latorre *et al.* 2001) are depicted in Fig. 9.1 on p. 122.

Interpretation of Fig. 9.5

- *QRS rate*: no QRS complexes present.
- *QRS rhythm*: no QRS complexes present.
- *QRS complexes*: no QRS complexes present.
- *P waves*: present.

- *Relationship between P waves and QRS complexes*: no QRS complexes present.

The ECG in Fig. 9.5 displays ventricular standstill. This patient was admitted with an extensive anterior myocardial infarction. Immediately prior to this episode of ventricular standstill, the ECG was displaying 2nd degree AV block type 2 (2:1 block). CPR was started and external pacing was instigated within minutes.

Interpretation of Fig. 9.6

- *QRS rate*: no QRS complexes present.

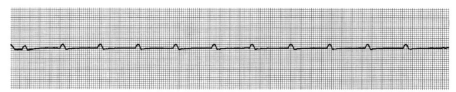

Fig. 9.5 Ventricular standstill

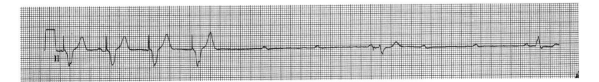

Fig. 9.6 Periods of ventricular standstill following ineffective transvenous pacing (due to malposition of pacing wire)

- *QRS rhythm*: no QRS complexes present.
- *QRS complexes*: no QRS complexes present.
- *P waves*: present.
- *Relationship between P waves and QRS complexes*: no relationship.

The ECG in Fig. 9.6 displays ventricular standstill. This patient had a temporary transvenous cardiac pacemaker inserted for 3rd degree AV block following an anterior myocardial infarction. Unfortunately it became ineffective due to malposition, resulting in ventricular standstill. External pacing was applied until the temporary transvenous pacing wire could be repositioned.

PULSELESS ELECTRICAL ACTIVITY

Pulseless electrical activity (PEA) is the presenting rhythm in approximately 35% of in-hospital cardiac arrests (Gwinnutt *et al.* 2000). PEA (formally called electromechanical dissociation or EMD) is a term used when there is no cardiac output, despite the presence of a normal (or near-normal) ECG. PEA can be classified as either primary or secondary.

Primary PEA is caused by a failure of excitation contraction coupling in the cardiac cells causes a profound loss of cardiac output. Causes include massive myocardial infarction, poisoning and electrolyte imbalance. Secondary PEA is caused by a mechanical barrier to ventricular filling or ejection. Causes include cardiac tamponade, tension pneumothorax, pulmonary embolism and hypovolaemia. In all cases, treatment is directed at the cause.

Identifying features on the ECG
The ECG trace displayed is normal or near-normal (Colquhoun & Camm 1999). The patient could be in a state of cardiac arrest despite monitoring sinus rhythm.

Effects on the patient
The patient will have a cardiac arrest.

Treatment
Confirm cardiac arrest and start CPR. Treatment is aimed at identifying and treating the cause if possible.

The European Resuscitation Council guidelines for the management of pulseless electrical activity (non-VF/VT) (Latorre *et al.* 2001) are depicted in Fig. 9.1.

AGONAL RHYTHM
Agonal rhythm is characterised by slow, irregular, wide QRS complexes of varying morphology (Resuscitation Council UK 2000). It is commonly described as the 'dying heart rhythm' and can be seen towards the end of an unsuccessful CPR attempt. True stimulation of the myocardium does not occur and it may continue for several minutes despite the patient being clinically dead (Meltzer *et al.* 1983). The rate slows down until asystole ensues.

Identifying features on the ECG

- *QRS rate*: usually very slow (< 30/min).
- *QRS rhythm*: irregular.
- *QRS complexes*: very wide and bizarre.
- *P waves*: absent.
- *Relationship between P waves and QRS complexes*: unable to determine.

Effects on the patient
The patient will already have had a cardiac arrest.

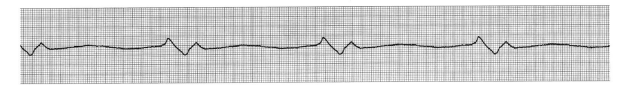

Fig. 9.7 Agonal rhythm

Treatment
CPR will usually be stopped.

Interpretation of Fig. 9.7

- *QRS rate*: 25.
- *QRS rhythm*: regular.
- *QRS complexes*: very wide and bizarre.
- *P waves*: absent.
- *Relationship between P waves and QRS complexes*: no P waves present.

CHAPTER SUMMARY
Cardiac arrhythmias associated with cardiac arrest have been discussed in this chapter. These include ventricular fibrillation (VF), pulseless ventricular tachycardia (VT), asystole, ventricular standstill, pulseless electrical activity (formally called electromechanical dissociation or EMD) and agonal rhythm.

REFERENCES

Bradbury, N., Hyde, D. & Nolan, J. (2000) Reliability of ECG monitoring with a gel pad/paddle combination after defibrillation. *Resuscitation* **44**: 203–6.

Chamberlain, D. (1999) Spurious asystole with use of manual defibrillators. *British Medical Journal* **319**: 1574.

Cobbe, S., Redmond, M., Watson, J. *et al.* (1991) Heartstart Scotland – initial experience of a national scheme for out of hospital defibrillation. *British Medical Journal* **302**: 1517– 20.

Colquhoun, M., Camm, A. (1999) Asystole and electromechanical dissociation, in Colquhoun, M., Handley, A. & Evans, T. (eds) *ABC of Resuscitation*, 4th edn. BMJ Books, London.

Colquhoun, M. & Chamberlain, D. (1999) Ventricular fibrillation, in Colquhoun, M., Handley, A. & Evans, T. (eds) *ABC of Resuscitation*, 4th edn. BMJ Books, London.

Colquhoun, M. & Jevon, P. (2000) *Resuscitation in Primary Care*. Butterworth Heinemann, Oxford.

Gwinnutt, C., Columb, M. & Harris, R. (2000) Outcome after cardiac arrest in adults in UK hospitals: effect of the 1997 guidelines. *Resuscitation* **47**: 125–35.

Jevon, P. (2002) *Advanced Cardiac Life Support*. Butterworth Heinemann, Oxford.

Kerber, R. & Robertson, C. (1996) Transthoracic defibrillation, in Paradis, N., Halperin, H., Nowak, R. (eds) *Cardiac Arrest: The Science and Practice of Resuscitation Medicine*. Williams & Wilkins, London.

Larsen, M., Eisenberg, M., Cummins, R. & Hallstrom, A. (1993) Predicting survival from out-of-hospital cardiac arrest: a graphic model. *Annals of Emergency Medicine* **22**: 85–91.

Latorre, F., Nolan, J., Robertson, C. *et al.* (2001) European Resuscitation Council Guidelines 2000 for adult advanced life support. *Resuscitation* **48**: 211–21.

McWilliam, J. (1889) Cardiac failure and sudden death. *British Medical Journal* Jan. **5**: 6–8.

Mapin, D., Brown, C. & Dzuonczyk, R. (1991) Frequency analysis of the human and swine electrocardiogram during ventricular fibrillation. *Resuscitation* **22**: 85–91.

Meltzer, L.E., Pinneo, R. & Kitchell, J.R. (1983) *Intensive Coronary Care: A Manual for Nurses*, 4th edn. Prentice Hall, London.

Resuscitation Council UK (2000) *Advanced Life Support Manual*, 4th edn. Resuscitation Council UK, London.

Sedgwick, M., Dalziel, K., Watson, J. *et al.* (1994) The causative rhythm in out-of-hospital cardiac arrests witnessed by the emergency medical services in the Heartstart Scotland project. *Resuscitation* **27**: 55–9.

Recording a 12 Lead ECG

10

INTRODUCTION

An electrocardiograph (Fig. 10.1) is a machine that records the waveforms generated by the heart's electrical activity. An electrocardiogram (ECG) is the collection of electrical waveforms produced.

The recording of a 12 lead ECG must be undertaken meticulously. Care should taken to ensure accuracy and standardisation: poor technique can lead to misinterpretation of the ECG, mistaken diagnosis, wasted investigations and mismanagement of the patient. To quote Marriott (1988): 'heart disease of electrocardiographic origin should be avoided'.

The aim of this chapter is to understand the principles of recording a 12 lead ECG.

LEARNING OBJECTIVES

At the end of the chapter the reader will be able to:

❏ list the common indications for recording a 12 lead ECG;

❏ describe a procedure for recording a standard 12 lead ECG;

❏ discuss how to ensure accuracy, quality and standardisation when recording a 12 lead ECG;

❏ discuss what the standard 12 lead ECG records.

COMMON INDICATIONS FOR RECORDING A 12 LEAD ECG

Common indications for recording a 12 lead ECG include:

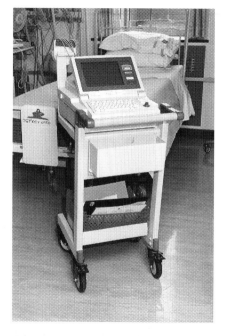

Fig. 10.1 Electrocardiograph or ECG machine

- chest pain;
- myocardial infarction;
- sometimes prior to a general anaesthetic;
- cardiac arrhythmias;
- palpitations;
- history of syncope;
- post successful CPR.

PROCEDURE FOR RECORDING A STANDARD 12 LEAD ECG

A suggested procedure for recording a standard 12 lead ECG is:

(1) Identify the patient.
(2) Explain the procedure to the patient.
(3) Assemble the equipment. It is important to ensure that the ECG cables are not twisted as this can cause interference (Metcalfe 2000).
(4) Ensure the environment is warm and the patient is relaxed as much as possible. This will help produce a clear, stable trace without interference.

(5) Ensure the patient is lying down in a comfortable position, ideally resting against a pillow at an angle of 45 degrees with the head well supported (identical patient position should be adopted as with previous 12 lead ECGs: this will help ensure standardisation). The inner aspects of the wrists should be close to, but not touching, the patient's waist.

(6) Prepare the skin if necessary. If wet gel electrodes are used, shaving and abrading the skin is not required. If solid gel electrodes are used, clean/degrease and debrade the skin and shave if necessary.

(7) Apply the electrodes (Fig. 10.2) and the limb leads:
 (a) red to the inner right wrist;
 (b) yellow to the inner left wrist;
 (c) black to the inner right leg, just above the ankle;
 (d) green to the inner left leg, just above the ankle.

(8) Apply the electrodes to the chest (Figs 10.3 and 10.4) and attach the chest leads:

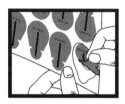

Fig. **10.2** ECG electrodes (reproduced by kind permission of Medicotest, manufacturer of 'blue sensor electrodes')

 (a) V1 (white/red lead): 4th intercostal space, just to the right of the sternum;
 (b) V2 (white/yellow lead): 4th intercostal space, just to the left of the sternum;
 (c) V3 (white/green lead): midway between V2 and V4;
 (d) V4 (white/brown lead): 5th intercostal space, mid-clavicular line;
 (e) V5 (white/black lead): on anterior axillary line, on the same horizontal line as V4;
 (f) V6 (white/violet lead): mid-axillary line, on the same horizontal line as V4 and V5.

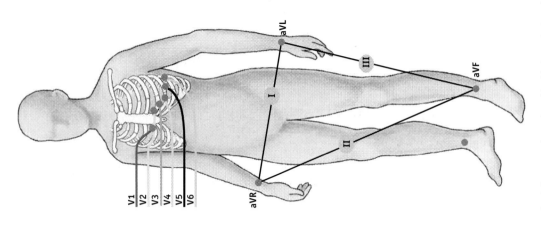

Fig. 10.3 Chest lead placement (reproduced by kind permission of Medicotest, manufacturer of 'blue sensor electrodes')

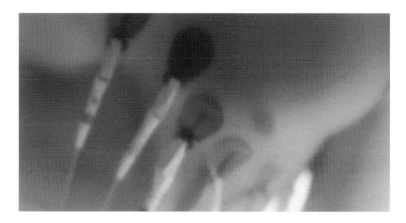

Fig. 10.4 Placement of chest leads on the chest (reproduced by kind permission of Medicotest, manufacturer of 'blue sensor electrodes')

(9) Check the calibration signal on the ECG machine to ensure standardisation (Metcalfe 2000).

(10) Ask the patient to lie still and breathe normally.

(11) Print out the ECG following the manufacturer's recommendations.

(12) Once an adequate 12 lead ECG has been recorded, disconnect the patient from the ECG machine and clear equipment away and clean as necessary following the manufacturer's recommendations. Sometimes electrodes are left on

the patient if serial recordings are going to be required.

(13) Ensure the ECG is correctly labelled. Report and store the ECG in the correct patient's notes following local procedures.

Locating the intercostal spaces for the chest leads

Using the right clavicle as a reference to palpate the 1st intercostal space can lead to mistaking the space between the clavicle and the 1st rib as the 1st intercostal space. It is therefore recommended to use the angle of Louis as a reference point for locating the 2nd intercostal space. The procedure is:

(1) palpate the angle of Louis (sternal angle) – it is at the junction between the manubrium and the body of the sternum;

(2) slide the fingers towards the right side of the patient's chest and locate the 2nd rib, which is attached to the angle of Louis;

(3) slide the fingers down towards the patient's feet and locate the 2nd intercostal space;

(4) slide the fingers further down to locate the 3rd and 4th ribs and the corresponding four intercostal spaces.

Alternative chest lead placements

Alternative chest lead placements are sometimes indicated:

- *Right-sided*: inferior or posterior myocardial infarction, to ascertain whether there is right ventricular involvement (these patients may require careful management for hypotension and pain relief) and dextrocardia. The chest leads are labelled V3R to V6R and are in effect reflections of the left-sided chest leads V3 to V6.

- *Posterior*: particularly if there are reciprocal changes

in V1–V2, suggesting posterior myocardial infarction. Chest leads are applied to the patient's back below the left scapula, corresponding to the same level as the 5th intercostal space, to view the posterior surface of the heart.

- *Higher or more lateral on the chest*: if the clinical history is suggestive of myocardial infarction, but the ECG is inconclusive.

Labelling the 12 lead ECG

Labelling the 12 lead ECG should follow local protocols (often done electronically). All relevant information should be included, i.e. patient details (name, unit number, date of birth), date and time of recording, ECG serial number together with any relevant information, e.g. if the patient was free from pain or complaining of chest pain during the recording, post-thrombolysis. The leads should be correctly labelled and deviations to the standard recording of a 12 lead ECG should be noted, e.g. right-sided chest leads, paper speed of 50 mm/s, different patient position.

ENSURING ACCURACY, QUALITY AND STANDARDISATION WHEN RECORDING A 12 LEAD ECG

Many variables can influence the recording of a 12 lead ECG trace without introducing unnecessary technical ones (Marriott 1988). Deviations from the standard procedure for the recording of a 12 lead ECG can lead to misinterpretation and misdiagnosis. It is therefore important to ensure accuracy, quality and standardisation when recording a 12 lead ECG.

Accuracy

Errors in electrode connection or placement are common (Jowett & Thompson 1995). Slight displacement of the chest leads can produce considerable changes in the ECG pattern (Marriott 1988). Interchanging limb leads could result in serious misinterpretation of the ECG, e.g. interchanged right arm and left leg leads produces a pattern mimicking inferior myocardial infarction with aVF resembling aVR.

Quality

Poor electrode contact, patient movement and electrical interference, e.g. from infusion pumps by the bed, can cause a fuzzy appearance on the ECG trace. Efforts should be made to minimise interference, ensure good electrode contact and relax the patient.

Standardisation

- To help comparison of serial 12 lead ECGs, they should be recorded with the patient in the same position. If this is not possible, e.g. if the patient has orthopnea, a note to this affect should be made because the electrical axis of the heart (main direct of current flow) can be altered which makes reviewing and comparing serial ECGs difficult (Marriott 1988).
- Standard calibration is 1 mV = 10 mm vertical deflection on the ECG (Fig. 10.5). If calibration varies from

recording to recording, ECG changes can sometimes be difficult to detect and the interpreter has to take into account inconsistencies in standardisation (Marriott 1988).
- Standard paper speed is 25 mm/s.

NB Any deviations to the standard procedure for the recording of a 12 lead ECG should be highlighted on the ECG. This will help to avoid possible misinterpretation and misdiagnosis.

WHAT THE STANDARD 12 LEAD ECG RECORDS

The heart generates electrical forces, which travel in multiple directions simultaneously. If the flow of current is recorded in several planes, a comprehensive view of this electrical activity can be obtained.

The standard 12 lead ECG records the electrical activity of the heart from 12 different viewpoints or leads ('leads' are viewpoints of the heart's electrical activity, they do not refer to the cables or wires which connect the patient to the monitor or ECG machine) by attaching 10 leads to the patient's limbs and chest.

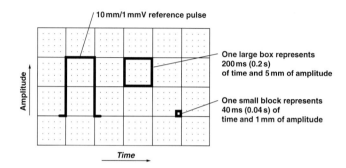

Fig. 10.5 Standard calibration (reproduced by kind permission of Medtronic)

Limb leads

If leads are attached to the patient's right arm, left arm and left foot, the three major planes for detecting electrical activity can be recorded (a fourth lead, attached to the right leg serves as a ground (earth) electrode and is not used for recording). A hypothetical triangle (Einthoven's triangle) is formed by these three planes, with the heart in the middle (Fig. 10.6).

These three different views of the heart are designated standard leads I, II and III (Jowett & Thompson 1995) and each records the difference in electrical forces between the two lead sites (Meltzer *et al.* 1983), hence the term bipolar leads. This electrode placement also permits recording from three unipolar leads: aVR, aVL and aVF.

Frontal plane

Bipolar leads

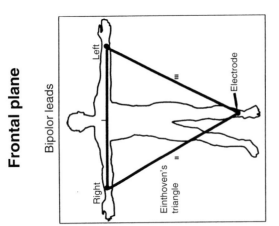

Left

Right

Electrode

III

II

Einthoven's
triangle

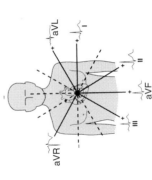

aVL

I

II

aVF

III

aVR

Fig. 10.6 Einthoven's triangle (reproduced by kind permission of Philips and Medtronic)

Chest leads

The six chest leads view the heart in a horizontal plane from the front (anterior) and from the side (lateral) (Fig. 10.7).

Standard placement of limb and chest leads and their relation to the surface of the heart

- Inferior surface of the heart: leads II, III, aVF.
- Anterior surface of the heart: leads V1, V2, V3, V4.
- Lateral surface of the heart: leads I, aVF, V5, V6.
- Septum: leads V2, V3.

Configuration of the ECG waveform

Electrical current flows between two poles, a positive (+) one and a negative (−) one. An upward deflection will be recorded on the ECG when the current is flowing towards the positive pole; whereas a downward deflection will be recorded if the current is flowing away from the positive pole.

If an impulse is travelling towards a lead then the QRS complex in that lead will be predominantly

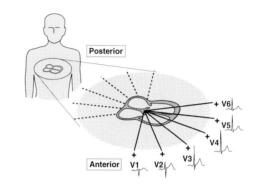

Fig. 10.7 Horizontal plane (chest leads) (reproduced by kind permission of Medtronic)

positive, whereas if it is moving away from the lead it will be predominantly negative.

During depolarisation of the intraventricular septum, the impulse travels initially from left to right (Fig. 10.8). The impulse then travels down the bundle branches and Purkinje fibres resulting in

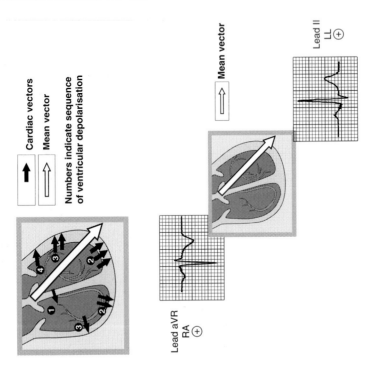

Cardiac vectors

Mean vector

**Numbers indicate sequence
of ventricular depolarisation**

Mean vector

Lead II
LL ⊕

Lead aVR
RA ⊕

Fig. 10.8 Mean vector of electrical activity (reproduced by kind permission of Medtronic)

multidirectional and simultaneous ventricular depolarisation (Fig. 10.8). In normal circumstances, the overall direction of depolarisation is towards the dominant mass of the left ventricle (Fig. 10.8). This results in:

- small Q waves and tall R waves in leads facing the left ventricle, e.g. leads II, V5, V6;
- small R waves and deep S waves in leads facing the right ventricle, e.g. V1, V2 (Fig. 10.8);
- R and S waves of equal size when the wave of depolarisation is at right angles to the lead, e.g. aVL.

Consequently the configuration of the ECG waveform will depend upon the ECG lead being monitored. Figures 10.9 and 10.10 depict typical ECG configurations in the limb and chest leads respectively.

CHAPTER SUMMARY
The 12 lead ECG is an essential diagnostic tool in the management of heart disease, in particular acute myocardial infraction. When recording a 12 lead ECG,

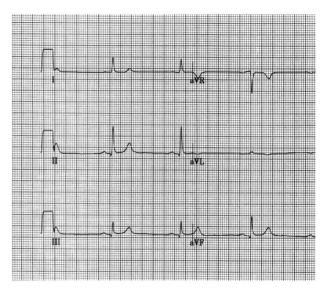

Fig. 10.9 Typical ECG configuration in the limb leads

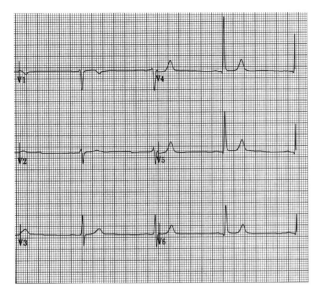

Fig. 10.10 Typical ECG configuration in the chest leads

care should be taken to ensure accuracy and standardisation in order to avoid possible misinterpretation of the ECG and mismanagement of the patient.

REFERENCES

Jowett, N.I. & Thompson, D.R. (1995) *Comprehensive Coronary Care* 2nd edn. Scutari Press, London.

Marriott, H.J.L. (1988) *Practical Electrocardiography*, 8th edn. Williams & Wilkins, London.

Meltzer, L.E., Pinneo, R. & Kitchell, J.R. (1983) *Intensive Coronary Care: A Manual for Nurses*, 4th edn. Prentice Hall, London.

Metcalfe, H. (2000) Recording a 12 lead electrocardiogram – 3. *Nursing Times* **96**(22): 45–6.

Interpreting a 12 Lead ECG

INTRODUCTION

The 12 lead ECG is an essential diagnostic tool in the management of heart disease. In particular, with the advent of thrombolytic therapy, the 12 lead ECG plays an important role in the early diagnosis of acute myocardial infarction. In addition it can provide detailed and useful information when interpreting of cardiac arrhythmias. When interpreting it in light of clinical history, the ECG can be invaluable in aiding selection of the most appropriate management (Channer & Morris 2002).

The aim of this chapter is to understand the principles of interpreting a 12 lead ECG.

LEARNING OBJECTIVES

At the end of the chapter the reader will be able to:

❏ describe a systematic approach to the interpretation of a 12 lead ECG;
❏ discuss the ECG features associated with myocardial infarction;
❏ discuss the ECG changes associated with bundle branch block;
❏ interpret a selection of 12 lead ECGs.

SYSTEMATIC APPROACH TO THE INTERPRETATION OF A 12 LEAD ECG

A systematic approach to the interpretation of a 12 lead ECG involves examining/checking:

- patient and ECG details;
- calibration;
- P waves;

145

- PR interval;
- QRS rate;
- QRS rhythm;
- QRS complexes;
- T waves;
- ST segment;
- QT interval;
- U waves;
- relationship between the P waves and QRS complexes;
- the rhythm;
- electrical axis;
- previous ECGs.

Patient and ECG details

Check the patient details: name, hospital number etc. Also check the ECG details including date and time of recording and whether there were any deviations to the standard approach to the recording of a 12 lead ECG.

Calibration

Check the calibration of the ECG (see Fig. 10.5 in Chapter 10).

P waves

Establish whether P waves are present. If they are present determine the rate and whether their morphology is normal and constant.

As atrial activation spreads across the atria in an inferior direction towards the AV junction, P waves are usually upright in leads facing the inferior surface of the heart (leads II, III and aVF) and inverted in aVR which faces the superior surface.

Changes in P wave morphology implies a different pacemaker focus for the impulse. Retrograde activation through the AV junction (junctional or ventricular arrhythmias) usually results in the P waves being inverted in leads II, III and aVF (atrial depolarisation opposite direction to normal).

The amplitude should not exceed 3 mm, the width (duration) should not exceed 0.11 s/2.75 small squares and the shape should be round, not notched or pointed. When examining P waves it is important to look for the following abnormalities:

- *Increased amplitude* (> 3mm): usually indicative of atrial hypertrophy or dilation. Often associated with hypertension or AV valve disease.
- *Increased duration* (> 0.11s): usually indicative of left atrial enlargement.
- *Inversion in leads when normally upright*: inverted P waves in leads I and II are indicative of the spread of the impulse across the atria in an unorthodox way, e.g. APB, JPB.
- *Notching*: left atrial enlargement sometimes referred to as P mitrale.
- *Peak complex*: tall, pointed P waves, more noticeable in lead III than in lead I, resulting from right atrial overload, sometimes referred to as P-pulmonale.
- *Diphasicity*: when the second part of the P wave is significantly negative in lead III or V1, it is an important sign of left atrial enlargement.

Sometimes it may be difficult to establish whether P waves are present because they are partly or totally obscured by the QRS complexes or T waves, e.g. in sinus tachycardia P waves may merge with the preceding T waves.

In SA block and sinus arrest, P waves will be absent. In atrial fibrillation, no P waves can be identified, just a fluctuating baseline. In atrial flutter, P waves are replaced by regular sawtooth flutter waves, rate approximately 300/min.

PR interval

Calculate the PR interval. It represents the time taken for the impulse to travel from the SA node to the ventricles. It is measured from the beginning of the P wave to the beginning of the QRS complex. The normal PR interval is 0.12–0.20s (3–5 small squares). It varies with heart rate: the faster the heart rate, the shorter the interval.

A prolonged PR interval (> 0.20s) is indicative of AV block. Sometimes it is a normal variation. A shortened

PR interval (< 0.12s) is associated with an AV junctional pacemaker or the presence of an accessory pathway, e.g. Wolff–Parkinson–White syndrome.

QRS rate

Estimate the QRS rate by counting the number of large (1 cm) squares between two adjacent QRS complexes and dividing it into 300 (caution if the QRS rate is irregular). For example, the QRS rate in Fig. 3.2 in Chapter 3 is about 75/min (300/4).

An alternative method is to count the number of QRS complexes in a defined number of seconds and then calculate the rate per minute. For example, if there are 12 QRS complexes in a 10s strip; ventricular rate is 72/min (12×6).

- Normal QRS rate: 60–100/min.
- Slow QRS rate (bradycardia): < 60/min.
- Fast QRS rate (tachycardia): > 100/min.

NB A pulse rate of 50 may be 'normal' in some patients and one of 70 may be abnormally slow in other patients.

QRS rhythm

Ascertain whether the QRS rhythm is regular or irregular. Using the rhythm strip displayed on the ECG, carefully compare RR intervals. Callipers may help.

Alternatively plot two QRS complexes on a piece of paper. Then move the paper to other sections on the rhythm strip and ascertain whether the marks are aligned exactly with other pairs of QRS complexes (regular QRS rhythm) or not (irregular QRS rhythm).

If the QRS rhythm is found to be irregular, determine whether it is totally irregular or whether there is a cyclical variation in the RR intervals (Resuscitation Council UK 2000).

A totally irregular QRS rhythm is most likely going to be atrial fibrillation, particularly if the morphology of the QRS complexes remains constant. If there is a cyclical pattern to the irregularity of the RR intervals, examine the relationship between the P waves and QRS complexes (see below). The presence of ectopics can render an otherwise regular QRS rhythm irregular.

Determine whether they are atrial, junctional or ventricular.

QRS complexes

Examine the morphology of the QRS complexes. The QRS complex represents the spread of the impulse through the ventricles and is labelled as follows:

- Q wave: if the first deflection of the complex is negative or downward.
- R wave: the first positive or upright deflection.
- S wave: negative deflection following an R wave.
- R1: if there is a second positive deflection.
- S1: if there is a second negative deflection.

Lower case and capital letters are used to describe the relative sizes of the QRS components.

When examining the morphology of the QRS complexes, measure the width and amplitude and examine any Q waves.

Width

Normal width is < 0.12 s/3 small squares. A QRS width of 0.12 s/3 small squares or more is indicative of abnormal intraventricular conduction, either bundle branch block or a ventricular arrhythmia.

If the patient has a tachyarrhythmia with a wide QRS complex, it is important to establish whether it is supraventricular or ventricular in origin. Supraventricular tachyardia with aberration (i.e. impulses are conducted to the ventricles with bundle branch block resulting in wide QRS complexes) can mimic ventricular tachycardia. Most wide complex tachycardias are ventricular in origin. According to Marriott (1988), the following ECG features favour ventricular origin:

- R or qR (rabbit ear) in V1;
- rS or QS in V6;
- all QRS complexes in the chest leads either positive or negative;
- extreme axis deviation (−90° to −180°) – positive aVR;

- QRS complex > 0.14 s/3.5 small squares;
- presence of fusion beats and/or capture beats;
- AV dissociation.

Again according to Marriott (1988), the following ECG features favour aberrant conduction:

- rsR morphology in V1;
- qRs morphology in V6;
- QRS morphology identical to pre-existing bundle branch block;
- if there is right bundle branch block and the initial QRS deflection is identical to that with the normal beats.

Amplitude (voltage)

The total amplitude, i.e. above and below the isoelectric line, should be greater than 5 mm in the standard limb leads. Abnormally low voltage may be seen in pericardial effusion, myxoedema and widespread myocardial damage. The distance the recording leads are away from the heart can also influence the voltage – chest size, chest wall thickness etc. should be taken into account when examining the amplitude.

Ventricular hypertrophy will result in increased electrical activity and an increase in height of the QRS complex. In right ventricular hypertrophy, the lead facing the right ventricle (V1) displays dominant R waves (at least 5 mm tall) instead of the usual dominant S waves (Julian & Cowan 1993). In left ventricular hypertrophy, the leads facing the left ventricle (V5 and V6) display tall R waves (> 25 mm) and the lead facing the right ventricle (V1) displays deep S waves.

Q waves

Small narrow Q waves are normal in leads facing the left ventricle, i.e lead I, aVL, aVF, V5 and V6. Wide (> 0.04 s/1 small square) and deep (> 2 mm) Q waves are indicative of myocardial infarction (Hampton 2000). The presence of Q waves in lead III is sometimes a normal finding.

T waves

Examine the T waves. They represent repolarisation of the ventricles. Note the direction, shape and height. They are normally upright in leads I, II and V3–V6, inverted in aVR and variable in the other leads. They are normally slightly rounded and asymmetrical. Their height should not be > 5 mm in the standard leads or > 10 mm in the chest leads.

Sharply pointed T waves is suggestive of myocardial infarction or hyperkalaemia. Notched T waves are sometimes found in pericarditis. Inverted T waves can be associated with myocardial ischaemia, digoxin toxicity and ventricular hypertrophy.

The T wave morphology can be affected by myocardial ischaemia in a variety of different ways: tall, flattened, inverted or biphasic (Channer & Morris 2002).

In ventricular hypertrophy the T waves are inverted and asymmetrical (Julian & Cowan 1993). In left ventricular hypertrophy, the T waves are inverted in the left ventricular leads, i.e. leads II, aVL, V5 and V6; in right ventricular hypertrophy, the T waves are inverted in the right ventricular leads, i.e. V2 and V3 (Hampton 2000).

ST segment

Examine the ST segment. It represents the period following ventricular depolarisation (end of QRS complex) to the beginning of ventricular repolarisation (beginning of the T wave). It is usually isoelectric. Note the level of the ST segment in relation to the baseline (elevation or depression) and also its shape.

Elevation or depression is indicative of an abnormality in the onset of ventricular muscle recovery. Elevation > 1 mm in the limb leads and > 2 mm in the chest leads is abnormal. The commonest causes of ST segment elevation is myocardial infarction. Widespread (and not localised) ST segment elevation (concave upwards) is characteristic of pericarditis. ST segment elevation is sometimes a normal finding in healthy young black men (Marriott 1988).

The ST segment shape should gently curve into the T wave. Depression > 0.5 mm is abnormal (Julian &

Cowan 1993). Horizontal depression of the ST segment, together with an upright T wave, is usually indicative of myocardial ischaemia (Hampton 2000). In digoxin toxicity, the ST segment is down-sloping or sagging (Channer & Morris 2002), particularly prominent in leads II and III.

QT interval

Calculate the QT interval. It represents the total duration of ventricular depolarisation and repolarisation. It is measured from the beginning of the QRS complex to the end of the T wave. It varies with heart rate, sex (longer in women) and age. The normal QT interval is usually less than half of the preceding RR interval (Marriott 1988) and the upper limit of normal is 0.40 s / 2 large squares (Hampton 2000).

A prolonged QT interval indicates that ventricular repolarisation is delayed, which could result in the development of tachyarrhythmias. Causes of a prolonged QT interval include drugs, hypothermia and electrolyte imbalance.

U waves

U waves are low voltage waves that may be seen following the T waves. Their source is uncertain (Marriott 1988). They share the same polarity as the T waves and are best viewed in V3. They are more prominent in hypokalaemia.

Relationship between the P waves and QRS complexes

Establish whether the P waves and QRS complexes are 'married' to each other. Ascertain whether each P wave is followed by a QRS complex and each QRS complex is preceded by a P wave.

If the PR interval is constant, atrial and ventricular activity is likely to be associated. If the PR interval is variable, establish whether atrial and ventricular activity is associated or dissociated. Map out the P waves and QRS complexes and examine their relationship. Look for any recognisable patterns, the presence of dropped beats and PR intervals that vary in a repeated fashion (Resuscitation Council UK 2000).

AV dissociation is when the atria and ventricles are depolarised by two different sources. It is seen for example in 3rd degree AV block and sometimes in ventricular tachycardia. It is not a diagnosis in itself, but a clinical feature identified on the ECG of a cardiac arrhythmia.

Electrical axis

In order to depolarise every cardiac cell, the electrical impulses must travel in many different directions through the myocardium. These different directions of current flow collectively determine the electrical summation vector or axis during depolarisation and systole (Paul & Hebra 1998). Normally, the axis is down and to the patient's left, reflecting the impulse direction down from the SA node, through the AV junction and down to and through the ventricles (see Fig. 10.8 in Chapter 10).

For simplification, Marriott (1988) defines a normal axis as between 0 and 90°, right axis deviation as between +90° and +180°, and left axis deviation as between 0 and −90° (see Fig. 11.1).

There are several methods that can be used to calculate the cardiac axis; some are more confusing than others. Some basic principles to consider when calculating the electrical axis are as follows:

- The lead with the largest positive QRS deflection is the closest of the six limb leads towards which the electrical summation vector or axis travels.
- The lead with the largest negative QRS deflection is the furthest of the six limb leads away from which the electrical summation vector or axis travels.
- The electrical axis points towards leads whose R waves are larger than the S waves.
- The electrical axis points away from leads whose R waves are smaller than the S waves.
- The electrical axis is at right angles to the lead with equally sized R and S waves.

Houghton and Gray (1998) suggest the following quick and simple technique for working out the cardiac axis. Examine leads I and II. If the QRS complex is:

- predominantly positive in both leads I and II, the axis is normal;
- predominantly positive in lead I but predominantly negative in lead II, there is left axis deviation;
- predominantly negative in lead I, but predominantly positive in lead II, there is right axis deviation.

(For most practical purposes, it is not necessary to determine the exact axis of the heart.)

A useful aide-mémoire is:

- if lead I is predominantly positive and lead II is predominantly negative, they will be pointing away from each other, i.e. they have *left* each other – left axis deviation;
- if lead I is predominantly negative and lead II is predominantly positive, they will be pointing towards each other, i.e. they are *right* for each other – right axis deviation.

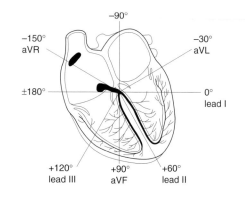

Fig. 11.1 Hexaxial reference system (reproduced by kind permission of Williams & Wilkins)

Causes of left axis deviation include:

- left bundle branch block;
- left anterior fasicular block;
- ventricular arrhythmias.

Causes of right axis deviation include:

- right bundle branch block;
- left posterior fasicular block;
- ventricular arrhythmias.

ECG CHANGES ASSOCIATED WITH MYOCARDIAL INFARCTION

Over 80% of patients with acute myocardial infarction present with an abnormal ECG (Jowett & Thompson 1995). However, less than 50% of patients initially present with typical and diagnostic ECG changes (Channer & Morris 2002). Sometimes the ECG may be normal or inconclusive. Nevertheless, despite some limitations, the ECG is probably still the best way of diagnosing myocardial infarction (Timmis 1990).

Daily (often subtle) ECG changes can be of major value in the diagnosis of myocardial infarction, especially when they are interpreted with the knowledge of the clinical history and serum enzyme changes (Jowett & Thompson 1995). Approximately 10% of patients with a proved myocardial infarction (clinical history and cardiac enzyme rises) fail to develop ST segment elevation or depression (Morris & Brady 2002).

Within minutes of myocardial infarction

Within minutes of myocardial infarction, the normal QRS complex (Fig. 11.2) with a tall R wave and a positive T wave, changes. The earliest signs are subtle: T waves over the affected area become more pronounced, symmetrical and pointed. These T waves, often referred to as 'hyperacute T waves', are more evident in the anterior leads and are more easily iden-

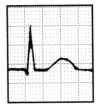

Fig. 11.2 Normal QRST complex (reproduced by kind permission of Medicotest, manufacturer of 'blue sensor electrodes')

tified if an old 12 lead ECG is available for comparison (Morris & Brady 2002).

These T wave changes are quickly followed by ST segment elevation (Fig. 11.3), which is often seen in leads facing the affected area of the myocardium. It is caused by damaged, but not necrosed, myocardial tissue. It can occur within minutes of the onset of chest pain and is a characteristic ECG change used as a criterion for the administration of thrombolytic therapy (Colquhoun 1993).

Hours to days following myocardial infarction

Hours to days following the event, in the leads facing the affected area, the R waves become smaller. Wide (> 0.04 s/1 small square) and deep (> 2 mm) Q waves develop (Hampton 2000). In addition, the ST elevation begins to subside and T waves become increasingly negative (Fig. 11.4).

The presence of deep and broad Q waves indicates there is necrosed myocardial tissue in the heart which the leads face. The Q waves actually represent electri-

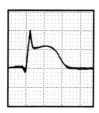

Fig. 11.3 ST segment elevation (reproduced by kind permission of Medicotest, manufacturer of 'blue sensor electrodes')

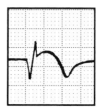

Fig. 11.4 ST segment begins to subside and T waves become increasingly negative (reproduced by kind permission of Medicotest, manufacturer of 'blue sensor electrodes')

cal activity in the opposite ventricular wall, which the leads view through an electrical window created by the necrosed (electrically inactive) myocardial tissue.

Days to weeks following myocardial infarction

Days to weeks later, the ST segment returns to the baseline and the T waves become more inverted and symmetrical (Fig. 11.5). Sometimes the R wave completely disappears.

Although most Q waves persist following a myocardial infarction, up to 15% can regress within 18

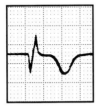

Fig. 11.5 Q waves and inverted T waves (reproduced by kind permission of Medicotest, manufacturer of 'blue sensor electrodes')

months with some ECGs returning to normal after 3 years (Surawicz *et al.* 1978).

Localising the myocardial infarction from the ECG

The characteristic changes seen in myocardial infarction are seen in the leads that record from the affected area. Familiarity with the areas of the myocardium represented by each of the ECG leads will enable not only the localisation of the infarction but also the extent of it. Common sites of infarction and the affected leads (Colquhoun 1993) are summarised as follows:

- inferior myocardial infarction: leads II, III, aVF;
- lateral myocardial infarction: leads I, aVL, V5, V6;
- anteroseptal myocardial infarction: V1, V2, V3;
- anterolateral myocardial infarction: V1, V2, V3, V4.

Right ventricular myocardial infarction, which is associated with 40% of inferior myocardial infarctions, is often overlooked because the standard 12 lead ECG does not provide a good indication of right ventricular damage (Morris & Brady 2002).

The presence of ST elevation in V1 does suggest right ventricular damage. However, right-sided chest leads (see page 136) are more sensitive and these should be recorded as soon as possible.

Q wave and non-Q wave infarctions

Q wave infarctions are commonly termed transmural or full-thickness infarctions. Non-Q wave infarctions are commonly termed not full-thickness or subendocardial infarctions. However, this pathology is often not correct (Hampton 2000).

In an extensive myocardial infarction, Q waves are a permanent sign of necrosis. However, when the myocardial infarction is more localised, the scar tissue may contract during the healing process, reducing the size of the electrically inert area resulting in the disappearance of the Q waves (Morris & Brady 2002).

Reciprocal changes

ST depression in leads remote from the site of the infarct are referred to as reciprocal changes. They are a highly sensitive indicator of acute myocardial infarction (Morris & Brady 2002). They may be seen in leads that do not directly view the affected area of myocardium (they reflect a mirror image of their opposite leads). In Fig. 11.6, ST elevation is evident in the inferior leads with reciprocal changes in the anterior leads. The depressed ST segments are typically horizontal or downsloping.

Reciprocal changes are seen in approximately 70% of inferior and 30% of anterior myocardial infarctions (Morris & Brady 2002). Reciprocal changes in the anterior chest leads V1–V3 are sometimes evident in a posterior myocardial infarction. The presence of reciprocal changes is particularly useful when there is doubt about the clinical significance of ST elevation (Morris & Brady 2002).

Diagnosing myocardial infarction in the presence of left bundle branch block

Diagnosing myocardial infarction in the presence of left bundle branch block can be very difficult. Q waves, ST segment and T wave changes can be obscured.

ECG examples of myocardial infarction

The ECG in Fig. 11.6 displays the characteristic ECG changes associated with acute inferior myocardial infarction. ST elevation can clearly be seen in leads II, III and aVF. Reciprocal changes can be seen, most markedly in lead aVL. Subsequent ECGs will probably indicate lateral involvement as well, i.e. inferolateral myocardial infarction. The ECG in Fig. 11.7, recorded with right-sided chest leads, displays right ventricular involvement. This patient was admitted with a one hour history of crushing central chest pain. The ECG changes are typical of an acute infarct.

The ECG in Fig. 11.8 displays the characteristic ECG changes associated with inferior myocardial infarction. There is ST elevation in the inferior leads (II, III and aVF). However, the T waves in these leads are beginning to become negative. This, with the development of Q waves in the inferior leads, is suggestive that the infarct is not acute. This patient was admitted with a 24 hour history of central chest pain.

The ECG in Fig. 11.9 displays the characteristic ECG changes associated with posterior myocardial infarction. Tall R waves and reciprocal changes in anterior leads V1 and V2 and reciprocal changes in the anterior leads I and aVL would suggest this diagnosis. Posterior wall chest leads would be required to help confirm diagnosis of posterior myocardial infarction.

The ECG in Fig. 11.10 displays the characteristic ECG changes associated with anteroseptal or septal myocardial infarction. There is ST elevation in leads aVL and V1–V4. In addition there is right bundle branch block and left anterior fascicular block (bifascicular block), a complication of septal infarction. Regarding the right bundle branch block the familiar rSR morphology has been replaced with QR morphology due to the infarction.

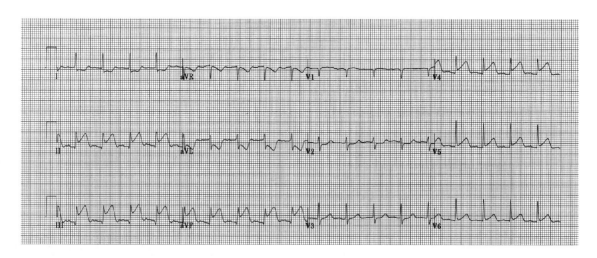

Fig. 11.6 Acute inferior myocardial infarction

The ECG in Fig. 11.11 displays the characteristic ECG changes associated with anteroseptal myocardial infarction. The abnormally tall and peaked T waves in leads V1–V4 are very suggestive of this. These ECG changes are hyperacute and are occasionally seen in the septal chest leads. This patient was admitted by his GP with a one hour history of chest pain.

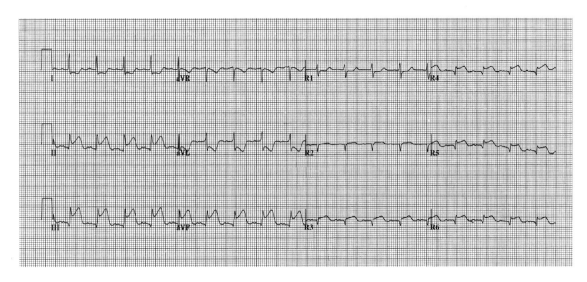

Fig. 11.7 Acute inferior myocardial infarction with right-sided chest leads indicating right ventricular involvement

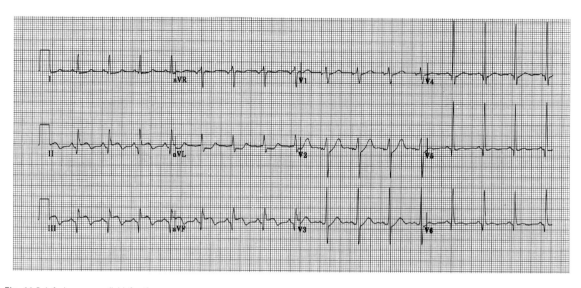

Fig. 11.8 Inferior myocardial infarction

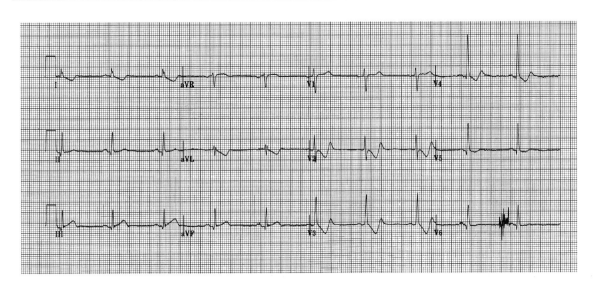

Fig. 11.9 Possible posterior myocardial infarction

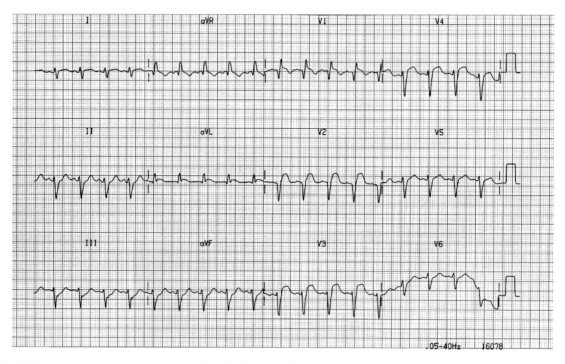

Fig. 11.10 Anteroseptal or septal myocardial infarction with bifascicular block

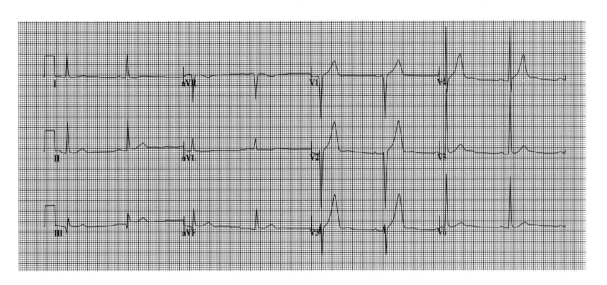

Fig. 11.11 Anteroseptal or septal myocardial infarction

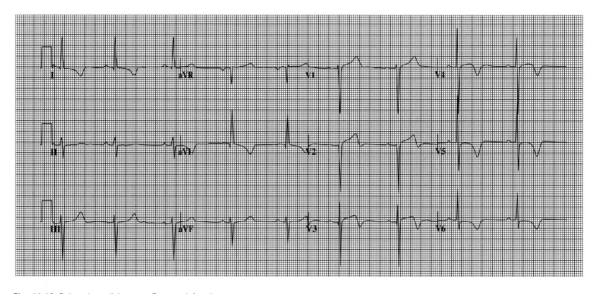

Fig. 11.12 Subendocardial or non-Q wave infarction

The ECG in Fig. 11.12 displays the characteristic ECG changes associated with subendocardial or the more commonly termed non-Q wave myocardial infarction. There is no loss of R waves or development of Q waves. However, there are abnormal changes in the T waves in the anterior leads I, aVL and V2–V6. Cardiac enzymes together with the patient's history will help confirm diagnosis.

ECG CHANGES ASSOCIATED WITH BUNDLE BRANCH BLOCK

Left bundle branch block

In left bundle branch block, conduction down the left bundle branches are blocked.

It is most commonly caused by ischaemic heart disease, hypertensive disease or dilated cardiomyopathy (Da Costa *et al*. 2002). It is rare for left bundle branch block to be present in the absence of organic disease (Da Costa *et al*. 2002).

Diagnosis can be made by examining chest leads V1 and V6:

- Septal depolarisation occurs from right to left: small Q wave in V1 and an R wave in V6 (the direction of intraventricular depolarisation is reversed, the septal waves are lost and are replaced with R waves) (Da Costa *et al*. 2002).
- Right ventricular depolarisation first: R wave in V1 and an S wave in V6 (often appearing as just a notch).
- Left ventricular depolarisation second: S wave in V1 and another R wave in V6.
- Delay in ventricular depolarisation leads to a wide (0.12 s/3 small squares or more) QRS complex.
- Abnormal depolarisation of the ventricles leads to secondary repolarisation changes: ST segment depression together with T wave inversion in leads with a dominant R wave; ST segment elevation and upright T waves in leads with a dominant S wave (i.e. discordance between the QRS complex and ST segment and T wave) (Da Costa *et al*. 2002).

Left bundle branch block is best viewed in V6: the QRS complex is wide and has an M-shaped configuration. The W-shaped QRS appearance in V1 is seldom seen.

The ECG in Fig. 11.13 displays left bundle branch block. The QRS width is 0.16 s/4 small squares. The W-shaped morphology of the QRS complex in V1 and the M-shaped morphology of the QRS complex in V6 can be seen clearly.

Right bundle branch block

In right bundle branch block, conduction down the right bundle branch is blocked. Conditions associated with right bundle branch block include ischaemic heart disease, pulmonary embolism, rheumatic heart disease and cardiomyopathy (Da Costa *et al.* 2002). Diagnosis can be made by examining chest leads V1 and V6:

- Septal depolarisation occurs from left to right as normal: small R wave in V1 and a small Q wave in V6.

- Left ventricular depolarisation first: S wave in V1 and an R wave in V6.
- Right ventricular depolarisation second: a second R wave in V1 and a deep wide S wave in V6.
- Latter part of the QRS complex is abnormal: slurred R and S waves in V1 and V6 respectively (Da Costa *et al.* 2002).
- ST segment depression and T wave inversion in the right precordial leads (Da Costa *et al.* 2002).

Right bundle branch block is best viewed in V1: the QRS complex is wide (0.12 s/3 small squares or more) and has a characteristic rSR pattern (see Fig. 11.14).

Left anterior fascicular block

In left anterior fascicular block (sometimes termed left anterior hemiblock), conduction down the anterior fascicle of the left bundle branch is blocked. Depolarisation of the left ventricle is via the left posterior fascicle. The cardiac axis therefore rotates in an upwards direction resulting in left axis deviation. Left anterior

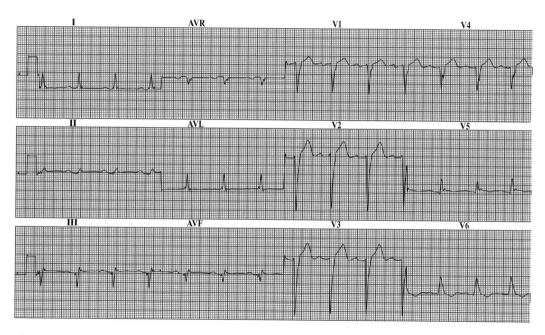

Fig. 11.13 Left bundle branch block

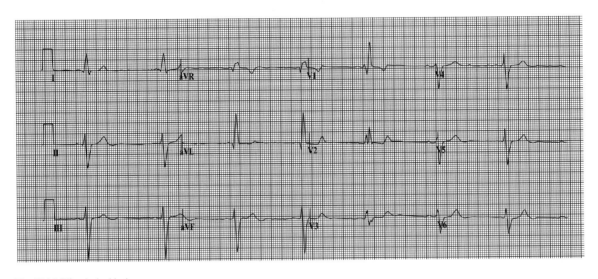

Fig. 11.14 Bifascicular block

fascicular block is characterised by a mean frontal plane axis more leftward than −30° in the absence of inferior myocardial infarction or other cause of left axis deviation (Da Costa *et al.* 2002).

Left posterior fascicular block

In left posterior fascicular block (sometimes termed left posterior hemiblock), conduction down the posterior fascicle of the left bundle branch is blocked. Depolarisation of the left ventricle is via the left anterior fascicle. The cardiac axis therefore rotates in a downwards direction resulting in right axis deviation.

Left posterior fascicular block is characterised by a mean frontal plane axis of greater than 90° in the absence of another cause of right axis deviation (Da Costa *et al.* 2002).

Bifascicular block

In bifascicular block, there is right bundle branch block and blockage of either the left anterior or posterior fascicle (determined by the presence of left or right axis deviation respectively). Right bundle branch block together with left anterior fascicular block is the commonest type of bifascicular block (Da Costa *et al.* 2002).

Bifascicular block is indicative of widespread conduction problems.

The ECG in Fig. 11.14 displays bifascicular block. There is right bundle branch block and left anterior fascicular block (left axis deviation).

Trifascicular block

Trifascicular block is when there is bifascicular block and first degree AV block (Da Costa *et al.* 2002). Third degree AV block will ensue if the other fascicle fails as well.

12 LEAD ECGS FOR INTERPRETATION

Figure 11.15 displays junctional tachycardia with associated widespread ST depression suggestive of myocardial ischaemia. This patient was complaining of chest pain and palpitations. Following the

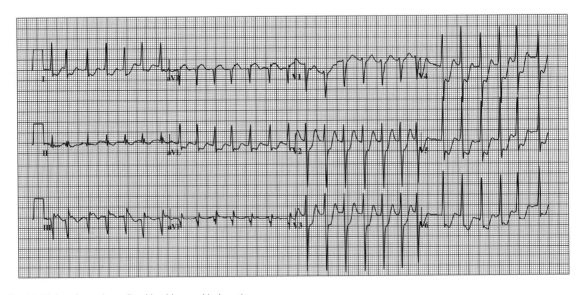

Fig. 11.15 Junction tachycardia with widespread ischaemia

administration of adenosine, the ECG reverted to sinus rhythm (Fig. 11.16). However, ST depression is still evident in the lateral leads (V4, V5 and V6). This patient required further investigations.

Figure 11.17 displays the characteristic ECG changes associated with inferolateral myocardial infarction with probable posterior involvement as well. There is ST elevation in leads II, III, aVF, V4, V5 and V6 (inferolateral). Tall R waves and reciprocal changes in V2 and V3 are suggestive of posterior involvement as well. Following the administration of diamorphine the ST elevation on the cardiac monitor settled. A repeat ECG (Fig. 11.18) was recorded which showed that the ST elevation had resolved. The diagnosis is probably Prinzmetal angina caused by transient coronary artery spasm.

Figure 11.19 displays atrial tachycardia with 2:1 AV block. The P waves are clearly visible in leads I, II and aVL. There are also pathological Q waves in leads II, III and aVF suggestive of an old inferior myocardial infarction.

Figure 11.20 displays atrial flutter with 3:1 AV block. The flutter waves are easily recognised in the inferior leads (II, III and aVF).

Figure 11.21 displays atrial flutter with 2:1 AV block resulting in a rapid ventricular response (approximately 160/min). The flutter waves can be clearly identified in lead aVR. The rate of the flutter waves is approximately 300/min, a distinguishable feature of atrial flutter. The atrial rate is too fast for atrial tachycardia.

Figure 11.22 displays junctional tachycardia. The narrow QRS complex is indicative of a supraventricular arrhythmia. Retrograde conducted P waves, a characteristic feature of a junctional arrhythmia, can clearly be identified in leads V1–V3.

Figure 11.23 displays ventricular tachycardia rate approximately 220/min. The QRS complexes are wide (> 0.12 s/3 small squares) and there is AV dissociation (P waves are clearly visible in the rhythm strip (calibration changed to help their identification). In addition there is right axis deviation (if the tachycardia

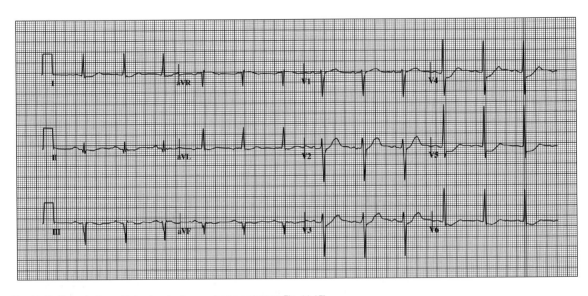

Fig. 11.16 Sinus rhythm with iscahemic changes (same patient as Fig. 11.15)

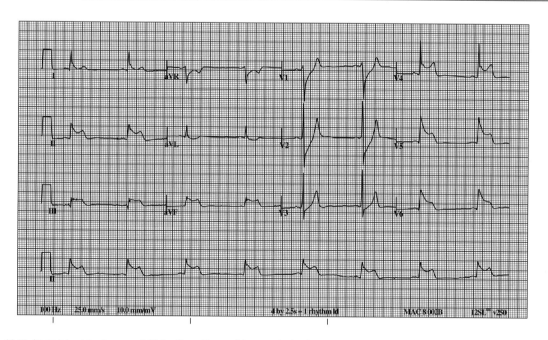

Fig. 11.17 Acute inferolateral myocardial infarction with possible posterior involvement, patient complaining of chest pain

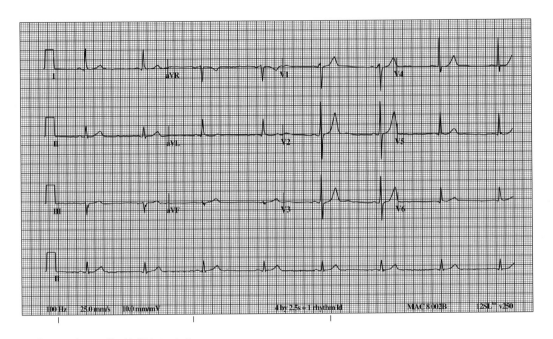

Fig. 11.18 Same patient as Fig. 11.17, but pain free

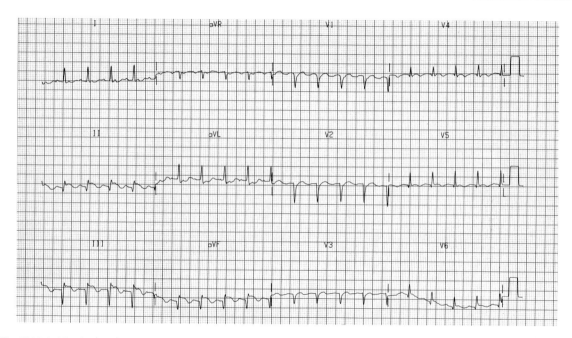

Fig. 11.19 Atrial tachycardia

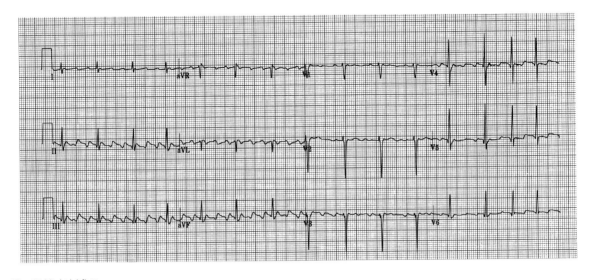

Fig. 11.20 Atrial flutter

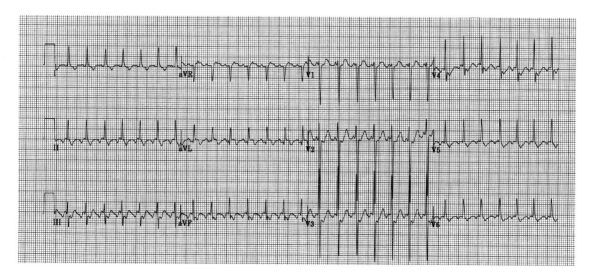

Fig. 11.21 Atrial flutter

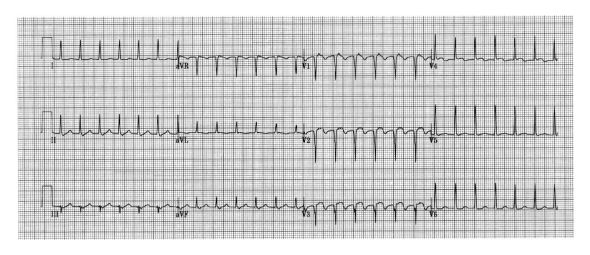

Fig. 11.22 Junctional tachycardia

was supraventricular in origin with left bundle branch block, then left axis deviation would be expected).

Figure 11.24 displays ventricular tachycardia. This is confirmed by a wide QRS complex (0.14 s/3.5 small squares), the presence of AV dissociation and the extreme left axis deviation with a positive aVR.

Figure 11.25 displays junctional tachycardia with aberration. There is borderline left bundle branch

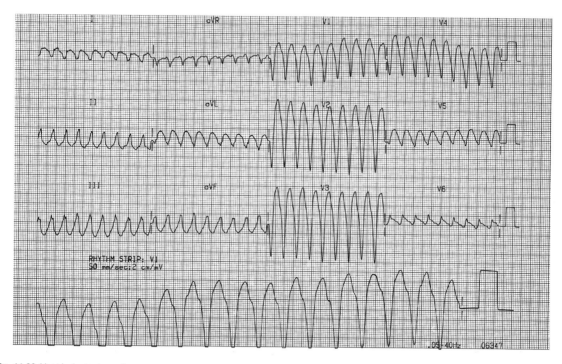

Fig. 11.23 Ventricular tachycardia

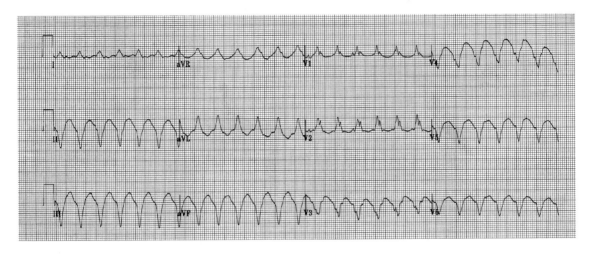

Fig. 11.24 Ventricular tachycardia

block pattern with a normal axis. No identifiable P waves.

Figure 11.26 displays left ventricular hypertrophy. Chest leads facing the left ventricle (V5 and V6) display abnormally tall R waves (> 25 mm) and inverted T waves. The chest lead facing the right ventricle (V1) displays an abnormally deep S wave (25 mm).

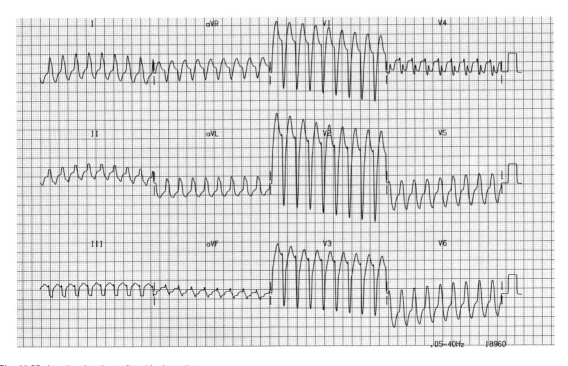

Fig. 11.25 Junctional tachycardia with aberration

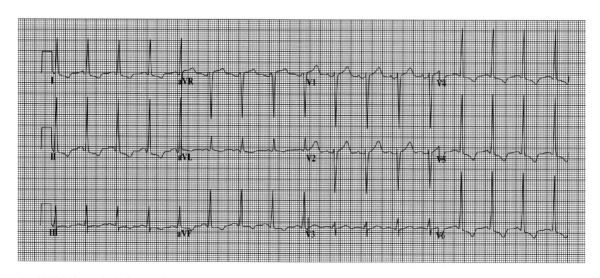

Fig. 11.26 Left ventricular hypertrophy

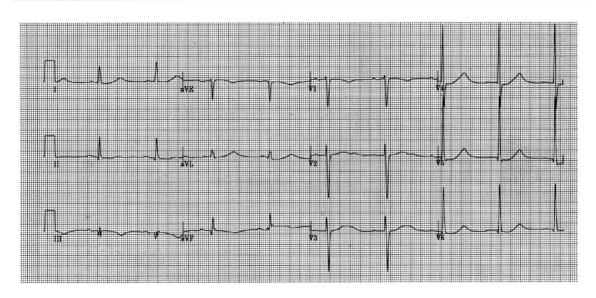

Fig. 11.27 Hypokalaemia

Figure 11.27 displays ECG changes associated with hypokalaemia. On close inspection, U waves can be identified in V2 and V3, which is characteristic of hypokalaemia. This patient's serum potassium was 2.6 mmol/litre.

CHAPTER SUMMARY

The 12 lead ECG is an essential diagnostic tool in the management of heart disease. In particular, with the advent of thrombolytic therapy, it plays an important role in the early diagnosis of acute myocardial infarction. When interpreting a 12 lead ECG it is important to follow a systematic and logical approach.

REFERENCES

Channer, K. & Morris, F. (2002) ABC of clinical electrocardiography: myocardial ischaemia. *British Medical Journal* **324**: 1023–6.

Colquhoun, M.C. (1993) *A Clinical Approach to Electrocardiography*. Napp Laboratories, Cambridge.

Da Costa, D., Brady, W. & Redhouse, J. (2002) ABC of clinical electrocardiography: bradycardias and atrioventricular block. *British Medical Journal* **324**: 535–8.

Hampton, J. (2000) *The ECG Made Easy*, 5th edn. Churchill Livingstone, London.

Houghton, A. & Gray, D. (1998) *Making Sense of the ECG*. Arnold, London.

Jowett, N.I. & Thompson, D.R. (1995) *Comprehensive Coronary Care*, 2nd edn. Scutari Press, London.

Julian, D. & Cowan, J. (1993) *Cardiology*, 6th edn. Baillière, London.

Marriott, H.J.L. (1988) *Practical Electrocardiography*, 8th edn. Williams & Wilkins, London.

Morris, F. & Brady, W. (2002) ABC of clinical electrocardiography: acute myocardial infarction – part 1. *British Medical Journal* **324**: 831–4.

Paul, S. & Hebra, J. (1998) *The Nurse's Guide to Cardiac Rhythm Interpretation*. W.B. Saunders, London.

Resuscitation Council UK (2000) *Advanced Life Support Manual*, 4th edn. Resuscitation Council UK, London.

Surawicz, B., Uhley, H., Borun, R. *et al.* (1978) Task force 1. Standardisation of terminology and interpretation. *American Journal of Cardiology* **41**: 130–45.

Timmis, A.D. (1990) Early diagnosis of acute myocardial infarction. *British Medical Journal* **301**: 941–2.

Treatment of Cardiac Arrhythmias

12

INTRODUCTION

The European Resuscitation Council's peri-arrest algorithms (Latorre *et al.* 2001) provide guidance for the treatment of bradycardia, narrow complex tachycardia, broad complex tachycardia and atrial fibrillation. Generally, a cardiac arrhythmia requires treatment only if it is serious, potentially serious or there are adverse signs. Sometimes it is possible to treat the underlying cause of the cardiac arrhythmia, e.g. electrolyte imbalance.

The aim of this chapter is to provide an overview of the treatment of cardiac arrhythmias. When reading this chapter it is important to read the text in conjunction with the European Resuscitation Council algorithms depicted in the chapter.

LEARNING OBJECTIVES

At the end of the chapter the reader will be able to:

❑ discuss the principles of using the European Resuscitation Council's peri-arrest algorithms;

❑ list the adverse clinical signs that may be associated with peri-arrest arrhythmias;

❑ discuss the treatment options;

❑ outline the management of bradycardia;

❑ outline the management of narrow complex tachycardia;

❑ outline the management of broad complex tachycardia;

❑ outline the management of atrial fibrillation;

❑ describe how to perform vagal manoeuvres;

❑ principles of synchronised cardioversion and defibrillation;

❑ discuss the key principles of cardiac pacing.

PRINCIPLES OF USING THE EUROPEAN RESUSCITATION COUNCIL'S PERI-ARREST ALGORITHMS

The European Resuscitation Council's peri-arrest algorithms (Latorre *et al.* 2001) are designed for the non-specialist as a guide, in the emergency situation, to provide effective and safe treatment of bradycardia, atrial fibrillation, narrow complex tachycardia and broad complex tachycardia (Jevon 2002). It is important to note that:

- they are specifically designed for the emergency situation and are not intended to encompass all clinical situations (Colquhoun & Vincent 1999);
- the arrows guide the practitioner from one stage of treatment to the next, only if the cardiac arrhythmia persists;
- the treatment of the patient is influenced by a number of variables including the arrhythmia itself, the patient's haemodynamic status, local procedures and circumstances;
- drug dose calculations are based on average body weight; adjustment may therefore be required in some situations;
- anti-arrhythmic strategies can be pro-arrhythmic;
- anti-arrhythmic drugs can cause hypotension and myocardial depression;
- if simple measures are ineffective, expert help should be summoned.

Jevon 2002

ADVERSE SIGNS ASSOCIATED WITH CARDIAC ARRHYTHMIAS

Adverse signs associated with cardiac arrhythmias include the following:

- *Clinical evidence of low cardiac output*, e.g. hypotension, pallor, cool peripheries and impaired consciousness caused by a fall in cerebral perfusion; the patient may become confused and agitated.

- *Excessive tachycardia*: narrow complex tachycardia > 200/min and broad complex tachycardia > 150/min can significantly reduce diastole, causing a decrease in coronary blood flow and myocardial ischaemia.
- *Excessive bradycardia*: usually < 40/min (higher rates may not be tolerated by some patients).
- *Cardiac failure*: pulmonary oedema, raised jugular venous pressure and hepatic engorgement (Resuscitation Council UK 2000) – these clinical features result from ineffective ventricular contraction.

Jevon 2002

TREATMENT OF BRADYCARDIA (FIG. 12.1)

By arbitrary definition, a ventricular rate of less than 60/min is defined as a bradycardia (Da Costa *et al.* 2002). However, rates above 60/min are inappropriately slow in some patients (relative bradycardia) (Colquhoun & Vincent 1999).

Management of the patient with a bradycardia is influenced by the presence or absence of symptoms and by whether treatment is likely to improve prognosis (Kishore *et al.* 1996).

Administer oxygen and secure i.v. access. If adverse signs (see above) are present, administer atropine. If there is no response to this and/or there is a risk of asystole, the definitive treatment is cardiac pacing. Interim measures include transcutaneous pacing or an epinephrine (adrenaline) infusion.

TREATMENT OF NARROW COMPLEX TACHYCARDIA (FIG. 12.2)

Intravenous access should be secured and oxygen administered. Provided there are no contraindications, vagal manoeuvres can be attempted, and if these fail, adenosine 6 mg administered i.v. If both of these interventions are unsuccessful and adverse signs are present, synchronised cardioversion is recommended.

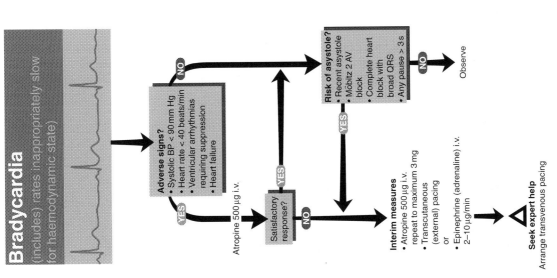

Bradycardia
(Includes) rates inappropriately slow
for haemodynamic state)

Adverse signs?
• Systolic BP < 90 mm Hg
• Heart rate < 40 beats/min
• Ventricular arrhythmias
  requiring suppression
• Heart failure

NO

YES

Atropine 500 µg i.v.

Satisfactory
response?

YES

NO

Risk of asystole?
• Recent asystole
• Möbitz 2 AV
  block
• Complete heart
  block with
  broad QRS
• Any pause > 3 s

YES

NO

Observe

Interim measures
• Atropine 500 µg i.v.
  repeat to maximum 3 mg
• Transcutaneous
  (external) pacing
or
• Epinephrine (adrenaline) i.v.
  2–10 µg/min

Seek expert help
Arrange transvenous pacing

Fig. 12.1 European Resuscitation Council guidelines for adult advanced life support: peri-arrest algorithm for bradycardia (reproduced by kind permission of Aurum pharmaceuticals)

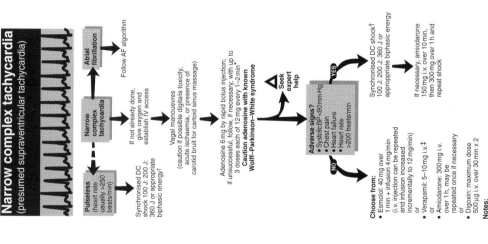

Narrow complex tachycardia
(presumed supraventricular tachycardia)

Pulseless
(heart rate usually >250 beats/min)

Synchronised DC shock 100 J: 200 J: 360 J or appropriate biphasic energy†

Narrow complex tachycardia

Atrial fibrillation

Follow AF algorithm

If not already done, give oxygen and establish IV access

Vagal manoeuvres
(caution if possible digitalis toxicity, acute ischaemia, or presence of carotid bruit for carotid sinus massage)

Adenosine 6 mg by rapid bolus injection; if unsuccessful, follow, if necessary, with up to 3 doses each of 12 mg every 1–2 min*
Caution adenosine with known Wolff–Parkinson–White syndrome

► **Seek expert help**

Adverse signs?
• Systolic BP <90 mm Hg
• Chest pain
• Heart failure
• Heart rate
  >200 beats/min

NO

Choose from:
• Esmolol: 40 mg over 1 min + infusion 4 mg/min (i.v. injection can be repeated and infusion increased incrementally to 12 mg/min)
or
• Verapamil: 5–10 mg i.v.‡
or
• Amiodarone: 300 mg i.v. over 1 h, may be repeated once if necessary
or
• Digoxin: maximum dose 500 μg i.v. over 30 min × 2

YES

Synchronised DC shock†
100 J: 200 J: 360 J or appropriate biphasic energy

If necessary, amiodarone 150 mg i.v. over 10 min, then 300 mg over 1 h and repeat shock

Notes:
A starting dose of 6 mg adenosine is currently outside the UK licence for this agent.
* Theophylline and related compounds block the effect of adenosine. Patients on dipyridamole, carbamazepine, or with denervated hearts have a marked exaggerated effect which may be hazardous.
† DC shock is always given under sedation/general anaesthesia.
‡ Not to be used in patients receiving beta-blockers.

Fig. 12.2 European Resuscitation Council guidelines for adult advanced life support: peri-arrest algorithm for narrow complex tachycardia (reproduced by kind permission of Aurum pharmaceuticals)

If there are no adverse signs, antiarrhythmic drugs such as amiodarone, verapamil or esmolol may be administered. If drugs fail, synchronised cardioversion may be required as a last resort.

TREATMENT OF BROAD COMPLEX TACHYCARDIA (FIG. 12.3)

Broad complex tachycardia will almost always be ventricular in origin (Colquhoun & Vincent 1999).

If the patient is pulseless, defibrillation is the definitive treatment (see Fig 9.1. in Chapter 9). If the patient has a pulse, but adverse signs are present, synchronised cardioversion should be undertaken, followed by amiodarone. Further synchronised cardioversion may be required. In refractory cases, amiodarone, lidocaine, procainamide or sotalol may be considered. Overdrive pacing is another option.

If there are no adverse signs, initial treatment options include amiodarone or lidocaine (lignocaine). Synchronised cardioversion may be required as a last resort. Correct any electrolyte imbalances.

TREATMENT OF ATRIAL FIBRILLATION (FIG. 12.4)

The treatment of atrial fibrillation is determined by whether it is low, intermediate or high risk.

High risk

Heart rate > 150/min, ongoing chest pain, critical perfusion.

The patient should be heparinised and then synchronised cardioversion undertaken as soon as possible. If synchronised cardioversion fails or if atrial fibrillation recurs, amiodarone should be administered before it is re-attempted.

Intermediate risk

Heart rate 100–150/min, dyspnoea, poor perfusion.

Treatment is determined by the patient's haemodynamic status, the duration of the atrial fibrillation arrhythmia and whether the patient has structural heart disease. There is a risk of an atrial thrombus developing in patients with atrial fibrillation of more than 24 hours.

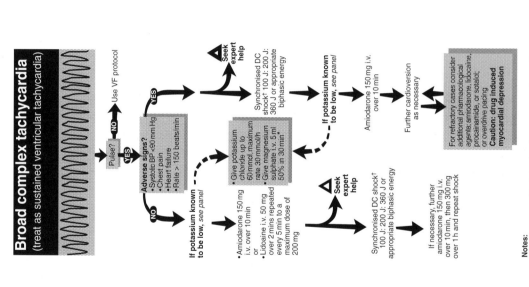

Broad complex tachycardia
(treat as sustained ventricular tachycardia)

Pulse? — NO → Use VF protocol

YES

Adverse signs?
• Systolic BP <90 mm Hg
• Chest pain
• Heart failure
• Rate > 150 beats/min

NO — YES

If potassium known to be low, *see panel*

• Amiodarone 150 mg i.v. over 10 min
or
• Lidocaine i.v. 50 mg over 2 mins repeated every 5 min to a maximum dose of 200 mg

⚠ Seek expert help

Synchronised DC shock† 100 J: 200 J: 360 J or appropriate biphasic energy

If necessary, further amiodarone 150 mg i.v. over 10 min, then 300 mg over 1h and repeat shock

• Give potassium chloride up to 60 mmol, maximum rate 30 mmol/h
• Give magnesium sulphate i.v. 5 ml 50% in 30 min*

⚠ Seek expert help

Synchronised DC shock† 100 J: 200 J: 360 J or appropriate biphasic energy

If potassium known to be low, *see panel*

Amiodarone 150 mg i.v. over 10 min

Further cardioversion as necessary

For refractory cases consider additional pharmacological agents: amiodarone, lidocaine, procainamide, or sotalol; or overdrive pacing
Caution: drug induced myocardial depression

Notes:
* *For paroxysms of torsades de points, use magnesium as above or overdrive pacing (expert help strongly recommended).*
† *DC shock is always given under sedation/general anaesthesia.*

Fig. 12.3 European Resuscitation Council guidelines for adult advanced life support: peri-arrest algorithm for broad complex tachycardia (reproduced by kind permission of Aurum pharmaceuticals)

194

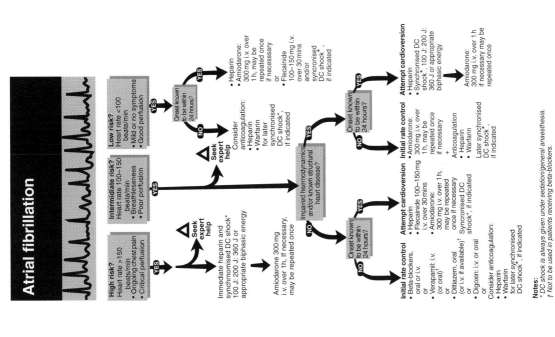

Atrial fibrillation

High risk?
- Heart rate >150 beats/min
- Ongoing chest pain
- Critical perfusion

Intermediate risk?
- Heart rate 100–150 beats/min
- Breathlessness
- Poor perfusion

Low risk?
- Heart rate <100 beats/min
- Mild or no symptoms
- Good perfusion

△ Seek expert help

Immediate heparin and synchronised DC shock* 100 J: 200 J: 360 J or appropriate biphasic energy

Amiodarone 300 mg i.v. over 1h, If necessary, may be repeated once

Impaired haemodynamics and/or known structural heart disease?

△ Seek expert help

Onset known to be within 24 hours? NO / YES

Initial rate control
- Beta-blockers, oral or i.v.
- or
- Verapamil i.v. (or oral)†
- or
- Diltiazem, oral (or i.v. if available)†
- or
- Digoxin: i.v. or oral
- or

Consider anticoagulation:
- Heparin
- Warfarin for later synchronised DC shock*, if indicated

Attempt cardioversion
- Heparin
- Flecainide 100–150mg i.v. over 30 mins
- Amiodarone: 300 mg i.v. over 1h, may be repeated once if necessary

Synchronised DC shock*, if indicated

Initial rate control
- Amiodarone: 300 mg i.v. over 1 h, may be repeated once if necessary

+ Anticoagulation
- Heparin
- Warfarin

Later synchronised DC shock*, if indicated

Onset known to be within 24 hours? NO / YES

Consider anticoagulation:
- Heparin
- Warfarin for later synchronised DC shock*, if indicated

Onset known to be within 24 hours? NO / YES

- Heparin
- Amiodarone: 300 mg i.v. over 1 h, may be repeated once if necessary
- or
- Flecainide 100–150mg i.v. over 30 mins and/or synchronised DC shock*, if indicated

Attempt cardioversion
- Heparin
- Synchronised DC shock*, 100 J: 200 J: 360 J or appropriate biphasic energy

Amiodarone: 300 mg i.v. over 1 h if necessary may be repeated once

Notes:
* DC shock is always given under sedation/general anaesthesia.
† Not to be used in patients receiving beta-blockers.

Fig. 12.4 European Resuscitation Council guidelines for adult advanced life support: peri-arrest algorithm for atrial fibrillation (reproduced by kind permission of Aurum pharmaceuticals)

- *No evidence of impaired haemodynamics or structural heart disease, but the onset of atrial fibrillation > 24 hours previously*: the ventricular rate should be controlled using drugs. Synchronised cardioversion should be performed only once the patient has being anti-coagulated for three/four weeks (Resuscitation Council UK 2000).

- *No evidence of impaired haemodynamics or structural heart disease, but the onset of atrial fibrillation < 24 hours previously*: the patient should be heparinised and restoration of sinus rhythm should be attempted, e.g. flecainide, amiodarone. Synchronised cardioversion may be needed.

- *Evidence of impaired haemodynamics and/or structural heart disease, but the onset of atrial fibrillation > 24 hours previously*: the ventricular rate should be controlled with amiodarone. Synchronised cardioversion should be attempted only once the patient has being anticoagulated for three/four weeks (Resuscitation Council UK 2000).

- *Evidence of impaired haemodynamics and/or structural heart disease, but the onset of atrial fibrillation < 24 hours previously*: the patient should be heparinised and synchronised cardioversion performed to restore sinus rhythm. Amiodarone may be required.

Low risk

Heart rate < 100/min, mild or no symptoms, good perfusion.

- *Onset of atrial fibrillation > 24 hours previously*: anti-coagulation should be considered and synchronised cardioversion performed after three/four weeks if required.

- *Onset of atrial fibrillation < 24 hours previously*: the patient should be heparinised and restoration of sinus rhythm should be attempted with either amiodarone or flecainide. Synchronised cardioversion may be required.

VAGAL MANOEUVRES

Vagal manoeuvres are used to stimulate the vagus nerve and induce a reflex slowing of the heart.

They can terminate narrow complex tachycardias in approximately 25% of cases (Resuscitation Council UK 2000).

Caution should be exercised regarding the use of vagal manoeuvres. Profound vagal tone can induce sudden bradycardia and trigger ventricular fibrillation, particularly in the presence of digitalis toxicity or acute cardiac ischaemia (Colquhoun & Vincent 1999).

Two vagal manoeuvres recommended by Colquhoun and Camm (1999) are carotid sinus massage and the Valsalva manoeuvre.

Carotid sinus massage

Carotid sinus massage is the most effective vagal manoeuvre (Mehta *et al.* 1988).

Unfortunately it is not risk free. It can cause rupture of an athermatous plaque, which could lead to cerebral embolism (Colquhoun & Camm 1999). It should therefore not be used if there is a recent history of transient cerebral ischaemia and should be used with extreme caution in the presence of a high-pitched carotid bruit (Thompson 1997). Elderly patients are more vulnerable to plaque rupture and cerebral vascular complications (Bastuli & Orlowski 1985; Skinner & Vincent 1997).

The procedure for carotid sinus massage as described by Thompson (1997) is as follows:

(1) Position the patient in a semi-recumbent position.
(2) Ensure cardiac monitoring is established.
(3) Tilt the patient's chin upwards and away from the side which is going to be massaged.
(4) Palpate the carotid bulb and press firmly postero-medially in a massaging motion for 3–5 seconds.
(5) If unsuccessful, repeat the procedure on the other side (separately, never at the same time).
(6) Continually monitor the patient's ECG.

Valsalva manoeuvre

The Valsalva manoeuvre (forced expiration against a closed glottis) can also be effective. Position the patient in a supine position and ask him to blow into a 20 ml syringe with enough force to try to push the plunger back (Resuscitation Council UK 2000).

CATHETER ABLATION THERAPY

Catheter ablation therapy using radiofrequency has revolutionised the management of cardiac arrhythmias. It involves creating scar tissue in the heart which can destroy a normal or abnormal electrical connection or focus (Davis 1997).

It is usually undertaken following diagnostic electrophysiology studies. Once the arrhythmia focus has been identified and confirmed, the catheter is inserted and advanced to the target site with the help of diagnostic electrode catheters and radiology. For most arrhythmias, success is immediately evident; for a few, further electrophysiology studies are required to ascertain if it has been successful (Davis 1997).

PRINCIPLES OF SYNCHRONISED CARDIOVERSION AND DEFIBRILLATION

Synchronised cardioversion is a reliable method of converting a tachyarrhythmia to a normal rhythm (Resuscitation Council UK 2000). Owing to the associated risks, it is generally undertaken only when pharmacological intervention has been unsuccessful or if there are associated adverse signs, e.g. chest pain, hypotension, reduced level of consciousness, rapid ventricular rate and dyspnoea.

The shock should be delivered on the R wave and not on the vulnerable T wave which could precipitate VF. This is accomplished by securing a reliable ECG trace (usually lead II) using the defibrillator monitor and by pressing the 'sync' (synchronised) button on the defibrillator. A dot or arrow should appear only on the R waves.

Complications of synchronised cardioversion include VF and cerebral embolism. If atrial fibrillation requires urgent synchronised cardioversion, immediate heparinisation is indicated (Resuscitation Council UK 2000).

Procedure for synchronised cardioversion

The following procedure for emergency synchronised cardioversion is based on Resuscitation Council UK (2000) recommendations:

(1) Attach the defibrillator's ECG leads and establish an accurate ECG trace. Lead II is usually selected.

(2) Activate the 'sync' button on the defibrillator.

(3) Check that only the R waves are being synchronised; a dot or an arrow should appear on each R wave and not on other parts of the ECG complex, e.g. tall T waves.

(4) Place defibrillation gel pads on the patient's chest, one just to the right of the sternum, below the right clavicle and the other level with the 5th left intercostal space in the anterior axillary line (V5–V6 position on the ECG).

(5) Select 100J on the defibrillator.

(6) Apply the defibrillator paddles firmly on the defibrillation pads. It is important to apply the paddles according to their namesakes, i.e. sternum to sternum and apex to apex.

(7) Press the 'charge' button on the paddles to charge the defibrillator and shout 'stand clear'.

(8) Perform a visual check of the area to ensure that all personnel are clear.

(9) Check the monitor to ensure that the patient is still in the tachyarrhythmia that requires synchronised cardioversion. Also check that the 'sync' button is still activated and is synchronising only on the R waves.

(10) Press both discharge buttons simultaneously to discharge the shock. There will be a slight delay (until the next R wave) between pressing the shock buttons and shock discharge.

Points to note

- Obtain the patient's consent if possible.
- Ensure CPR equipment is immediately available.
- Sedate the patient if not unconscious – ideally an anaesthetist should be present.

- Use recommended shock energy levels – 100J, 200J and 360J (or biphasic equivalent) (Latorre *et al.* 2001).
- Reactivate 'sync' button if further synchronised cardioversion. (**NB** On some defibrillators the 'sync' button will remain activated once pressed and therefore needs to be switched off if no longer required.)
- Exercise extreme caution in patients with atrial fibrillation (see pages 193, 196).

Defibrillation

Early defibrillation is indicated for ventricular fibrillation and pulseless ventricular tachycardia – the chances of success decline substantially (7–10%) for every minute it is delayed (Cobbe *et al.* 1991). The recommended shock energy is 200J, 200J and 360J (or biphasic equivalent). The 'sync' button is not activated.

The implantable cardioverter defibrillator (ICD) can be used in patients with recurrent life-threatening ventricular arrhythmias who have not responded to conventional treatment. Its use is associated with improved chances of survival (Resuscitation Council UK 2000).

The ICD is positioned in a similar position to permanent pacemakers and can provide override pacing, low-energy synchronised cardioversion, high-energy defibrillation and pacing for bradycardia (Causer & Connelly 1998).

If a patient with an ICD has a cardiac arrest, standard CPR can be carried out without any risks to the team. If the ICD discharges it will not be detected by those carrying out the CPR. If external defibrillation is indicated, the paddles should be placed 12–15 cm away from the unit (Resuscitation Council UK 2000).

PRINCIPLES OF CARDIAC PACING

Cardiac pacing is required when the heart's natural pacemaker is either too slow or unreliable and not responding to the pharmacological treatment recommended in the bradycardia algorithm (see page 192). Specific indications for cardiac pacing include:

- SA node dysfunction resulting in symptomatic bradycardia or pauses;
- 2nd degree AV block Mobitz type 2;
- 3rd degree AV block;
- ventricular standstill;
- tachyarrhythmias requiring suppression (overdrive pacing);
- prophylactically if drug therapy could induce bradyarrhythmias;
- following catheter ablation of the AV junction.

Cardiac pacing can be non-invasive or invasive.

Non-invasive cardiac pacing

- *Percussion pacing*: a series of gentle blows over the precordium, lateral to the lower left sternal edge, at a rate of 100/min (Resuscitation Council UK 2000). Ideal in the CPR situation if transcutaneous pacing is not immediately available.
- *Transcutaneous pacing*: external method of pacing which is quick and easy to establish. Ideal for the CPR situation. It buys times while temporary transvenous pacing is established.

Invasive cardiac pacing

- *Temporary transvenous pacing*: a pacing catheter is inserted into the right ventricle via the venous system and then connected to an external pulse generator. Can be used for transient conduction disturbances or sometimes prophylactically for anticipated cardiac arrhythmias. Occasionally used for overdrive pacing of tachyarrhythmias. Requires skill to establish and life-threatening complications can occur.
- *Permanent transvenous pacing*: required if there is a permanent conduction problem. Most permanent implantable pacemakers are capable of both atrial and ventricular pacing, thus achieving more physiological pacing (Colquhoun & Camm 1999). Some devices respond automatically to changes in physical activity.

CHAPTER SUMMARY

This chapter has provided an overview to the treatment of cardiac arrhythmias based on the European Resuscitation Council's peri-arrest algorithms (Latorre *et al.* 2001). The use of vagal manoeuvres, drug therapy, synchronised cardioversion, defibrillation, pacing and catheter ablation have been described. In general, a cardiac arrhythmia requires treatment only if it is serious, potentially serious or there are adverse signs.

REFERENCES

Bastuli, J. & Orlowski, J. (1985) Stroke as a complication of carotid sinus massage. *Critical Care Medicine* **13**: 869.

Causer, J. & Connelly, D. (1998) Implantable defibrillators for life-threatening ventricular arrhythmias. *British Medical Journal* **317**: 762–3.

Cobbe, S., Redmond, M. & Watson, J. *et al.* (1991) Heartstart Scotland – initial experience of a national scheme for out of hospital defibrillation. *British Medical Journal* **302**: 1517–20.

Colquhoun, M. & Camm, A. (1999) Asystole and electro-mechanical dissociation. In: Colquhoun, M., Handley, A., & Evans, T. (eds) *ABC of Resuscitation*, 4th ed. BMJ Books, London.

Colquhoun, M. & Vincent, R. (1999) Management of peri-arrest arrhythmias, in Colquhoun, M., Handley, A. & Evans, T. (eds) *ABC of Resuscitation*, 4th edn. BMJ Books, London.

Da Costa, D., Brady, W. & Redhouse, J. (2002) ABC of clinical electrocardiography: bradycardias and atrioventricular block. *British Medical Journal* **324**: 535–8.

Davis, M. (1997) Catheter ablation therapy of arrhythmias, in Thompson, P. (ed.) *Coronary Care Manual*. Churchill Livingstone, London.

Jevon, P. (2002) *Advanced Cardiac Life Support*. Butterworth Heinemann, Oxford.

Kishore, A., Camm, A. & Bennett, D. (1996) Cardiac pacing. In: Julian, D., *et al.* (eds) *Diseases of the Heart*, 2nd ed. W.B. Saunders, London.

Latorre, F., Nolan, J. & Robertson, C. *et al.* (2001) European Resuscitation Council Guidelines 2000 for adult advanced life support. *Resuscitation* **48**: 211–21.

Mehta, D., Wafa, S., Ward, D. & Camm, A. (1988) Reactive efficacy of various physical manoeuvres in termination of junctional tachycardia. *Lancet* **1**: 1181–5.

Resuscitation Council UK (2000) *Advanced Life Support Manual*, 4th edn. Resuscitation Council UK, London.

Skinner, D. & Vincent, R. (1997) *Cardiopulmonary Resuscitation*. Oxford University Press, Oxford.

Thompson, P. (1997) *Coronary Care Manual*. Churchill Livingstone, London.

Record Keeping

INTRODUCTION

An accurate written record detailing relevant information concerning cardiac monitoring and the recording of 12 lead ECGs is important. It forms an integral part of the nursing management of the patient and can help to protect the practitioner if defence of his or her actions is required. Most of the text in this chapter is based on the NBM's *Guidelines for Records and Record Keeping* (originally published by UKCC).

The aim of this chapter is to understand the principles of good record keeping.

LEARNING OBJECTIVES

At the end of the chapter the reader will be able to:

❏ discuss the importance of good record keeping;
❏ outline the principles of good record keeping;
❏ state what should be documented on a 12 lead ECG and on an ECG rhythm strip;
❏ outline the importance of auditing records;
❏ discuss the legal issues associated with record keeping.

THE IMPORTANCE OF GOOD RECORD KEEPING

'Record keeping is an integral part of nursing, midwifery and health visiting practice. It is a tool of professional practice and one which should help the care process. It is not separate from this process and it is not an optional extra to be fitted in if circumstances allow.'

(NMC 2003)

Good record keeping will help to protect the welfare of both the patient and practitioner by promoting:

- high standards of clinical care;
- continuity of care through better communication and dissemination of information between members of the interprofessional healthcare team;
- early detection of problems, such as changes in the patient's condition;
- an accurate account of treatment and care planning and delivery.

The quality of record keeping is also a reflection on the standard of nursing practice. Good record keeping is an indication that the practitioner is professional and skilled whereas poor record keeping often highlights wider problems with the individual's practice (NBM 2003).

PRINCIPLES OF GOOD RECORD KEEPING

There are a number of factors which underpin good record keeping. The patient's records should:

- be factual, consistent and accurate;
- be documented as soon as possible after the event;
- be consecutive and accurately dated, timed and signed (including a printed signature);
- provide current information on the care and condition of the patient;
- be documented clearly and in such a way that the text cannot be erased;
- have any alterations and additions dated, timed and signed; all original entries clearly legible;
- not include abbreviations, jargon, meaningless phrases, irrelevant speculation and offensive subjective statements;
- still be legible if photocopied;
- identify any problems identified and, most importantly, the action taken to rectify them.

Best practice – record keeping

Records must be:

- factual;
- legible;
- clear;
- concise;
- accurate;
- signed;
- timed;
- dated.

Drew *et al.* 2000

- patient's personal details, e.g. name, unit number, date of birth;
- date and time of recording, together with any relevant information, e.g. if the patient was complaining of chest pain during the recording, post-thrombolysis;
- the leads (limb and chest) are correctly labelled;
- if there are changes to the standard recording, e.g. right-sided chest leads, paper speed of 50 mm/s;
- the ECG is stored in the appropriate place in the patient's notes, in chronological order with other ECGs.

ECG rhythm strips will also need to be correctly labelled and filed in the patient's notes in a chronological order.

It is also important to ensure that an accurate record is made in the patient's notes. In particular it is important to include interventions and any response to the interventions.

WHAT SHOULD BE DOCUMENTED ON A 12 LEAD ECG AND ON AN ECG RHYTHM STRIP

It is important to record all the necessary information documented on the 12 lead ECG. In most situations this will be done electronically. However, the nurse should check that the following have been recorded:

THE IMPORTANCE OF AUDITING RECORDS

Audit can play an important role in ensuring quality of healthcare. In particular it can help improve the process of record keeping. By auditing records the standard can be evaluated and any areas for improvement and staff development identified. Audit tools should be developed at a local level to monitor the standards of record keeping.

Audit should primarily be aimed at serving the interests of the patient rather than the organisation (NMC 2003). A system of peer review may also be of value. Whatever audit system is used, the confidentiality of the patient information applies to audit just as it does to record keeping.

LEGAL ISSUES ASSOCIATED WITH RECORD KEEPING

The patient's records are occasionally called in evidence before a court of law, by the Health Service Commissioner or in order to investigate a complaint at a local level. Sometimes the UKCC's Professional Conduct Committee may request the patient's records when investigating complaints related to misconduct. Care plans, diaries and anything that makes reference to the patient's care may be required as evidence (UKCC 1998).

What constitutes a legal document is often a cause for concern. Any document requested by the court becomes a legal document (Dimond 1994), e.g. nursing records, medical records, X-rays, laboratory reports, observation charts; in fact any document which may be relevant to the case.

If any of the documents are missing, the writer of the records may be cross-examined as to the circumstances of their disappearance (Dimond 2002). 'Medical records are not proof of the truth of the facts stated in them but the maker of the records may be called to give evidence as to the truth as to what is contained in them' (Dimond 2002).

'The approach to record keeping which courts of law adopt tends to be that "if it not recorded, it has not been done"' (NMC 2003). Professional judgement is required when deciding what is relevant and what needs to be recorded, particularly if the patient's clinical condition is apparently unchanging and no record has been made of the care that has been delivered.

A registered nurse has both a professional and a legal duty of care. Consequently, when keeping records it is important to be able to demonstrate that:

- a comprehensive nursing assessment of the patient has been undertaken, including care that has been planned and provided;
- relevant information is included together with any measures that have been taken in response to changes in the patient's condition;
- the duty of care owed to the patient has been honoured and that no acts or omissions have compromised the patient's safety;
- arrangements have been made for ongoing care of the patient.

The registered nurse is also accountable for any delegation of record keeping to members of the inter-professional team who are not registered practitioners. For example, if record keeping is delegated to a pre-registration student nurse or a healthcare assistant, competence to perform the task must be ensured and adequate supervision provided. All such entries must be countersigned.

The Data Protection Act 1998 gives patients the right to access their manually held and computerised health records. Sometimes it is necessary to withhold information, if it could affect the physical or mental well-being of the patient or if it would breach another patient's confidentiality (NMC 2003). If the decision to withhold information is made, justification for doing so must be clearly recorded in the patient's notes.

CHAPTER SUMMARY

When undertaking cardiac monitoring or recording a 12 lead ECG, it is important to ensure good record keeping. Good record keeping is both the product of good teamwork and an important tool in promoting high quality healthcare.

REFERENCES

Dimond, B. (2002) *Legal Issues of Nursing*, 3rd edn. Pearson Education, London.

Drew, D., Jevon, P. & Raby, M. (2000) *Resuscitation of the Newborn*. Butterworth Heinemann, Oxford.

NMC (2003) *Guidelines for Records and Record Keeping*. NMC, London.

Index